MEDITERRANEAN PASTA RECIPES

QUICK AND EASY MOUTH WATERING RECIPES FOR EVERY OCCASION

SANDRA RAMOS

Mediterranean Pata Recipes

SANDRA RAMOS

Copyright - 2021 - All rights reserved.

The content contained within this book may not be reproduced, duplicated or transmitted without direct written permission from the author or the publisher.

Under no circumstances will any blame or legal responsibility be held against the publisher, or author, for any damages, reparation, or monetary loss due to the information contained within this book, either directly or indirectly.

Legal Notice:

This book is copyright protected. This book is only for personal use. You cannot amend, distribute, sell, use, quote or paraphrase any part, or the content within this book, without the consent of the author or publisher.

Disclaimer Notice:

Please note the information contained within this document is for educational and entertainment purposes only. All effort has been executed to present accurate, up to date, and reliable, complete information. No warranties of any kind are declared or implied.
Readers acknowledge that the author is not engaging in the rendering of legal, financial, medical or professional advice. The content within this book has been derived from various sources. Please consult a licensed professional before attempting any techniques outlined in this book.

By reading this document, the reader agrees that under no circumstances is the author responsible for any losses, direct or indirect, which are incurred as a result of the use of information contained within this document, including, but not limited to, - errors, omissions, or inaccuracies.

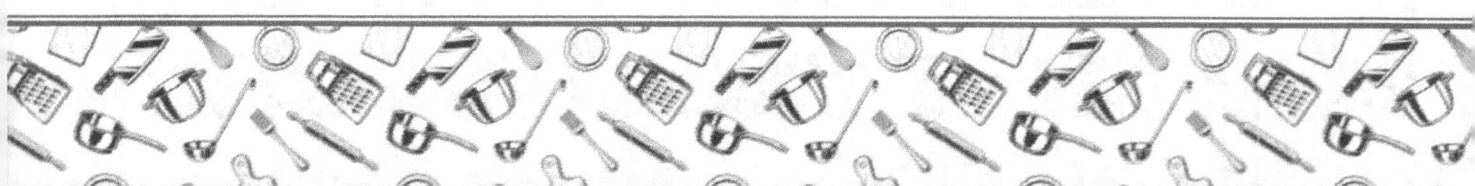

Table of Contents

INTRODUCTION 1

Chapter 1: Why this type of diet is the right for you? 5

Chapter 2: Your Mindset and this diet 9

Chapter 4: Exercise 15

Chapter 5: The recipes in this book 16

Pasta 18

    Simple Mac and Cheese Pasta 18

    Cold Spaghetti 19

    The Most Mediterranean Pasta Sauce 20

    Carbonara Spaghetti 21

    Penne with Asparagus and Shrimp 22

    Fettucine Lasagna 23

    Pasta with Lentil Soup 24

    Penne Key West 25

    Interesting Pasta 26

    Primavera from Cali 27

    Macaroni and Cheese vol.2 28

    Chicken and Tomato Pasta 29

    Pasta Bake with Vegetables and Cheese 30

    The Easiest Pasta on Earth 31

    Shrimp Pasta with Feta Cheese 32

Spaghetti Casserole	33
Pumpkin Pasta	34
Spaghetti Chicken	35
Pesto Pasta with Mint	36
Pasta Bake vol.2	37
Ham and Pea Spaghetti	38
Tuscan Style Pasta	39
Siciliano Pasta	40
Pomodoro Pasta	41
Basil and Tomato Pasta	42
Mac and Cheese vol.3	43
Rigatoni with Bean and Sausage	44
Penne, Goat Cheese and Arugula Pasta	45
Noodles vol.2	46
Basil and Red Pepper Pasta	47
Noodles from Poland	48
Taco Pasta	49
Shrimp Garlic Pasta	50
Tequila Pasta	51
Tortellini, Steak and Caesar	52
Ricotta Spaghetti	53
Salami and Bacon Spaghetti	54
Spinach and Feta Mostaccioli	55
Shrimp Garlic Pasta	56
Pasta and Spinach Shells	57

Fettucine Lasagna	58
Casserole from Pasta and Beans	59
Spinach and Feta Pasta	60
Lasagna with Mushrooms	61
Carbonara Spaghetti vol.1	62
Turkey Pasta	63
Fettuccine with Yogurt and Shrimp	64
Fagioli Pasta	65
Macaroni with 4 types of Cheese	66
Meatball and Pasta Dish	67
Spinach Noodles	68
Chicken Cacciatore and Pasta	69
Bow tie Pasta and Beef	70
4 of July Pasta	71
Chicken and Pasta with Balsamic Vinegar	72
Fettuccini Alfredo with Chicken	73
Manicotti	74
Cheddar Macaroni with Bacon and Thyme	75
Bang Noodles	76
Tarragon Chicken Pasta	77
Pasta with Vegetables, Tahini and Yogurt Sauce	78
Three Cheese Pasta	79
German Lasagna	80
Squash, Shrimp and Penne	81
Lasagna with Spinach and Cheese	82

- Lasagna with Artichokes and Spinach ... 83
- Basil Pasta ... 84
- Pasta and White Bean ... 85
- Pasta with Arugula Pesto ... 86
- Feta and Broccoli Pasta ... 87
- Her Highness – Pasta ... 88
- Shells with Bacon and Beef Sauce ... 89
- Bowties with Sausages and Artichokes ... 90
- Sausage Marinara Pasta ... 91
- Carbonara Fettucine ... 92
- Italian Macaroni and Cheese ... 93
- Cannoli ... 94
- The Easiest Lasagna Recipe on Earth ... 95
- Zucchini Pasta ... 96
- Meat Spaghetti ... 97
- Macaroni and Cheese Family Style ... 98
- Pasta Primavera without Cream ... 99
- Rigatoni in Vodka ... 100
- Pasta with Turkey ... 101
- Hudsucker Pasta ... 102
- Mostaccioli ... 103
- Chicken Manicotti ... 104
- Lamb Pasta ... 105
- Broccoli Lasagna ... 106
- Meat Spaghetti ... 107

Pizza Pie Pasta 108

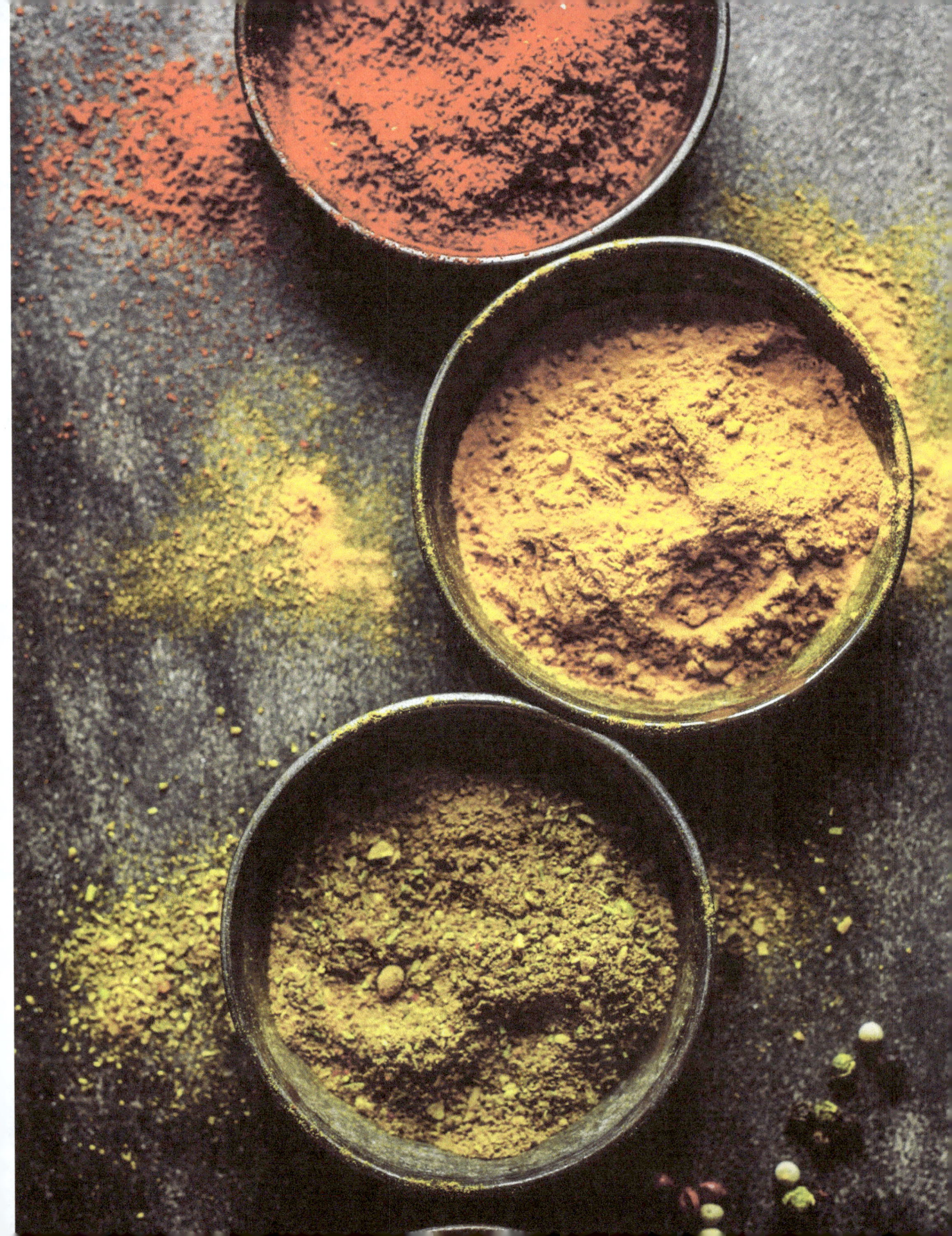

INTRODUCTION

The joy that I am feeling right now cannot be explained. This is because you have chosen me and this book as a guide to a new path – the Mediterranean one. The Mediterranean diet is like no other diet in this world and this way of eating is offering many health and weight benefits.

Right after World War II, Ancel Keys, a scientist and his colleague Paul Dudley, later known as President Eisenhower's cardiac physician made a Seven Countries Study together with couple of their colleagues. They included people from United States and people from Crete – Mediterranean island. The study was testing these people of all ages and Keys implemented the Mediterranean diet in this study as well.

The 13,000 men came from Netherlands, United States, Greece, Italy, Yugoslavia and Japan and it was estimated that fruits, vegetables, grains, beans and fish are the healthiest ingredients ever. This applies even after considering the impoverishment of WWII. Interestingly this was also estimated at the start, imagine what else they discovered.

Among everything else it was discovered that Mediterranean way of food consumption can make one person lose and maintain healthy weight. Every chapter included in this book will reveal different story about this diet plan and how can you become able to change your eating patterns. Also, you will find out that Mediterranean diet plan gives extreme amount of energy and you will become motivated

Chapter 1: Why this type of diet is the right for you?

Simply because it contains healthy plant foods and it is low in animal foods. Unlike other diets, Mediterranean diet offers more seafood and fish. Seafood and fish are way better than any other meat and the benefits of them is visible after a week or two of constant consumption. Plus, Mediterranean recipes do not leave you hungry, you are full after eating for a longer period.

With constant exercise and fruits, vegetables, legumes, nuts and whole grains (everything that this diet is) you will become the best version of yourself without doubt. Also, you will learn how to perfectly switch bad ingredients with good ingredients. For example, instead of butter you will start using canola or olive oil. Instead of salt you will start using different herbs and spices. Print out the Mediterranean pyramid of foods and you won't regret it.

These recipes are family friendly and you'll be able to host and enjoy and host many gatherings with your friends as well because they are also friend friendly. Occasional glass of red wine is okay, so you are good to go.

HEALTH BENEFITS

Healthy fats are the key component when it comes to Mediterranean cuisine. Also, let's not forget about the most important thing this diet has – plant-based food. Yes, this diet does not remove many food groups, but the mixture of ingredients won't make you a single problem and you will learn what goes with what in time.

But let's elaborate on the health benefits a little bit more. It is scientifically proven that the Mediterranean diet is able to lower the risk of strokes and heart disease. Every patient that has used this diet style so far, has shown lowered levels of oxidized low-density lipoprotein or LDL cholesterol (the bad cholesterol which gets build up in your arteries and causes problems with your heart.

NO MORE HEART PROBLEMS AND STROKES

One of the main ingredients in the Mediterranean diet, extra virgin olive oil, contains alpha-linolenic acid and the Warwick Medical School delivered a study that indicated how olive oil is able to decrease blood pressure. Not only that but also the olive oil is able to lower hypertension because it keeps human arteries clearer and more dilated. Also, it makes the nitric oxide more bioavailable and you won't have problems with cholesterol levels anymore. Only if of course, you consume olive oil (extra virgin) on regular bases.

If you are feeling numbness, weakness, headaches, confusion, vision problems, dizziness or slurred speech do not worry no more. This diet helps and improves this condition together with the ultimate problem – strokes that are happening due to bleeding in the brain or blocked blood vessel.

IMPROVED VISION

Another thing that would improve after starting with this diet is your vision. This diet will help you prevent or stave off the risk of macular degeneration which happens to adults over 54. This disease brings blindness and occurs to over 10 million Americans. Imagine the benefit in here, imagine being victorious against something that is able to destroy your retina and remove the chance of clear vision. The vegetables this diet promotes, the green leafy ones have lutein and that lowers the chance of experiencing cataracts as well.

WEIGHT LOSS

You probably want to lose weight as well and the search for the perfect diet that will be able to provide you that is endless. Until now. This diet is also able to give you the chance to lose weight naturally and easily with nutrient rich foods. The focus in here is on healthy fats while carbohydrates are not that present. They are still here as pasta or bread of course, but their implementation is generally low. The healthy fats, protein and fiber will allow you to lose weight and at the same time will keep you satisfied. Thanks to these nutrients you won't have cravings for candy, chips or cookies no more. The vegetables that you'll consume will fill your stomach and you won't feel hunger for hours. You won't even experience spike in your blood sugar.

IMPROVED AGILITY

According to studies, 70 percent of the seniors who have risk of developing frailty or other muscle weakness lowered the factors of experiencing that by implementing this diet in their lives.

YOU'LL START ENJOYING NATURAL FOODS

This is probably the best thing that this diet brings because it is kind of a new characteristic that you'll develop. As previously noted, this diet is low in sugar and processed foods so its recipes will bring you closer to organic produced foods thus closer to nature. For example, this diet offers honey instead of sugar and this change is priceless.

IMPROVED ASTHMA SYMPTOMS

Another study which included children revealed that antioxidant diet is able to help them decrease their asthma symptoms and at the same time made them not like eating a food that is quite popular – red meat. Yes, this diet helps children to say no to red meat and yes to plant-based food.

NO MORE ALZHEIMER'S RISK

Those people that choose this diet plant without doubt lower their risk of getting Alzheimer's disease in the future. In fact, the latest study shows that getting Alzheimer's is reduced by 40 percent to those people that consume Mediterranean diet foods. Additional exercises are recommended in the process as well.

HELPS PEOPLE WITH DIABETES

Excessive insulin is controlled with Mediterranean diet. Not every diet is able to do this and not every diet can control blood sugar levels and control your weight at the same time. As I told before this diet is at the same time low in sugar and high in healthy acids. This makes a balance for your body and burns fat while gives you energy at the same time.

The American Heart Association reveals that this diet unlike other diets is low in saturated fat while high in fat. This keeps your hunger under control and delivers amazing weight loss results.

MEDITERRANEAN DIET HELPS YOUR BRAIN

Sugar is usually responsible for the highs and lows when it comes to your mood. This diet does not contain artificial sugar at all this your mood and overall brain health will improve as well.

THE WEIGHT LOSS JOURNEY

Planning breakfast, lunch or dinner is not hard, but the part gets tricky when it comes to snacking time. You should make something for yourself that contains from 150 to 200 calories. For example, you can choose apple, pear, grapefruit and a pinch of salt.

The path that this diet offers is the safest when it comes to losing weight. Everything is healthy here and there won't be bouncing.

But many people ask what happens when the time is stumbling on us and when we do not have time to cook the meals present in here. Well, I and this diet of course have a solution for you. Trust me you will like it.

- Fruit slices – pears and apples
- Nut butter – cashew butter, almond butter and more
- Dates and figs
- Tuna salad
- Crackers
- Greek Yogurt
- Olives
- Pitas
- Hummus

Chapter 2: Your Mindset and this diet

In order to remove the unwanted pounds, you have to set your mindset on it like never before. Do not think about that all the time, start thinking about something entirely else while you are focused on losing weight. Or in other words, keep yourself busy while you consume Mediterranean diet foods and you regularly exercise. Also do not expect quick fixes. Time is all you need and after successfully sticking to the plant you'll start to realize the change and how big it is.

To be sincere, the Mediterranean diet is the one thing that you have been missing for so long. You are already motivated I think so all you have to do is start. You already purchased this book, so you are on the right path.

Write down your reasons for starting this journey and every time you are feeling down, or you lack motivated read them out loud. Write down your goals as well. Start with something small and increase as time passes.

Another important thing that people usually forget are their surroundings. It is important for you to surround with people that are positive. Positive mindset regardless of what you do is important, especially when it comes to losing weight and changing something as diet pattern. This is how you'll become able to develop emotionally, healthy realistic goals (do not forget to set your goals first).

Focus on your sleep and develop a healthy sleeping pattern as well. Recharging and sleeping for more than 7 hours are essential when it comes to weight loss because you need extreme amount of energy and sharpness. Good energy and brain sharpness appear only when one is able to properly relax and recharge in the evening hours.

Chapter 3: Nutrition and Portions

Start being aware of the things you consume now. Develop your management skills and stick to the guidelines that this book gives. What to consume? Well start with:

- Vegetables – raw and leafy
- Fruit
- Legumes
- Grains (one slice of bread is allowed)
- Dairy
- Meat
- Potatoes
- Nuts

This is the food you must start combining and portions that include these ingredients will make you set and ready for reaching your goals.

This is a sustainable diet so you won't have serious problems, but I will be lying if I say that cravings won't appear. If you successfully understand your cravings, you'll remove them and soon be proud of your dietary success. Remember, cravings for certain foods indicate need of something entirely else, something that your body is need of.

So, the adjustments that you have to make regarding the cravings are:

- Remove salty cravings with couple of nuts or seeds because your body want silicon.

- Remove fatty and oily foods with spinach, broccoli, cheese and fish because your body wants calcium and chloride.

- Remove sugary foods with chicken, beef, lamb, liver, cheese, cauliflower and broccoli because your body wants phosphorous and tryptophan.

- Remove chocolate cravings (this is the hardest one) with spinach, nuts, seeds, broccoli and cheese because your body wants magnesium and chromium.

You also have to:

- Learn how to recognize every healthy ingredient on the labels. Take back everything that does not look good to your or that indicates that there are many artificial preservatives present.

- Check your serving size.

- Always calculate your calories intake

- Consume food rich in calcium, iron, fiber, vitamin A and vitamin C.

Do not consume:

- Added sugar or foods like candy, soda, ice cream and more.

- Refined oils – soybean oil, canola oil cottonseed oil and more.

- Trans fats – margarine, soda, processed meats, beverages, table sugar and more.

- Processed meat.

- Refined grains.

Foods that you should consume:

- Seafood and Fish: Mussels, clams, crab, prawns, oysters, shrimp, tuna, mackerel, salmon, trout, sardines, anchovies, and more

- Poultry: Turkey, duck, chicken, and more

- Eggs: Duck, quail, and chicken eggs

- Dairy Products: Contain calcium, B12, and Vitamin A: Greek yogurt, regular yogurt, cheese, plus others

- Tubers: Yams, turnips, potatoes, sweet potatoes, etc.

- Vegetables: Another excellent choice for fiber, and antioxidants: Cucumbers, carrots, Brussels sprouts, tomatoes, onions, broccoli, cauliflower, spinach, kale, eggplant, artichokes, fennel, etc.

- Seedsand Nuts: Provide minerals, vitamins, fiber, and protein: Macadamia nuts, cashews, pumpkin seeds, sunflower seeds, hazelnuts, chestnuts, Brazil nuts, walnuts, almonds, pumpkin seeds, sesame, poppy, and more

- Fruits: Excellent choices for vitamin C, antioxidants, and fiber: Peaches, bananas, apples, figs, dates, pears, oranges, strawberries, melons, grapes, etc.

- Spices and Herbs: Cinnamon, garlic, pepper, nutmeg, rosemary, sage, mint, basil, parsley, etc.

- Whole Grains: Whole grain bread and pasta, buckwheat, whole wheat, barley, corn, whole oats, rye, quinoa, bulgur, couscous 18

- Legumes: Provide vitamins, fiber, carbohydrates, and protein: Chickpeas, pulses, beans, lentils, peanuts, peas

- Healthy Fats: Avocado oil, avocados, olive oil, olive oil products and olives

- Beverages: Water and tea

- White meat: Consume them but remove the visible fat and skin

- Red meat: You can consume lamb, pork, and beef in small amounts

- Potatoes: Prepare them with caution but consume them because they are excellent source of potassium, vitamin b, vitamin c and fibers.

- Desserts and sweets: consume cakes, biscuits and sweets in extra small amounts.

There is one thing that you can implement that will make your journey even more beautiful – spices and herbs! Traditional Mediterranean diet is filled with different spices and herbs and each has a different health benefit! Believe it or not herbs and spices are able to do that and that is one of the main reasons why people implement them in their diet. Here are the spices you must include and the benefits they bring:

- Anise – improves digestion, reduces nausea and alleviates cramps.

- Bay leaf – treats migraines.

- Basil – aids digestion and reduces anxiety and stress.

- Black pepper – promotes nutrient absorption and speeds up your metabolism.

- Cayenne pepper – increases metabolism and controls your appetite.

- Sweet and spicy cloves – relive pain, gum and tooth pain. Also, kill bacteria, fungal infections and aid digestive problems.

- Fennel – improves bone health.

- Garlic – improves blood sugar levels and helps you lose weight.

- Ginger – serves as diuretic and increases urine elimination.

- Marjoram – promotes healthy digestion and fights type 2 diabetes.

- Mint – treats nasal congestion, nausea, dizziness and headaches.

- Oregano – treats common cold and reduces infections. It also relieves menstrual pain.

- Parsley – improves your skin, prostate, dental health and blood circulation.

- Rosemary – increases hair growth, reduces stress, inflammation and improves pain.

- Sage – improves your digestion problems.

- Thyme – has antibacterial properties.

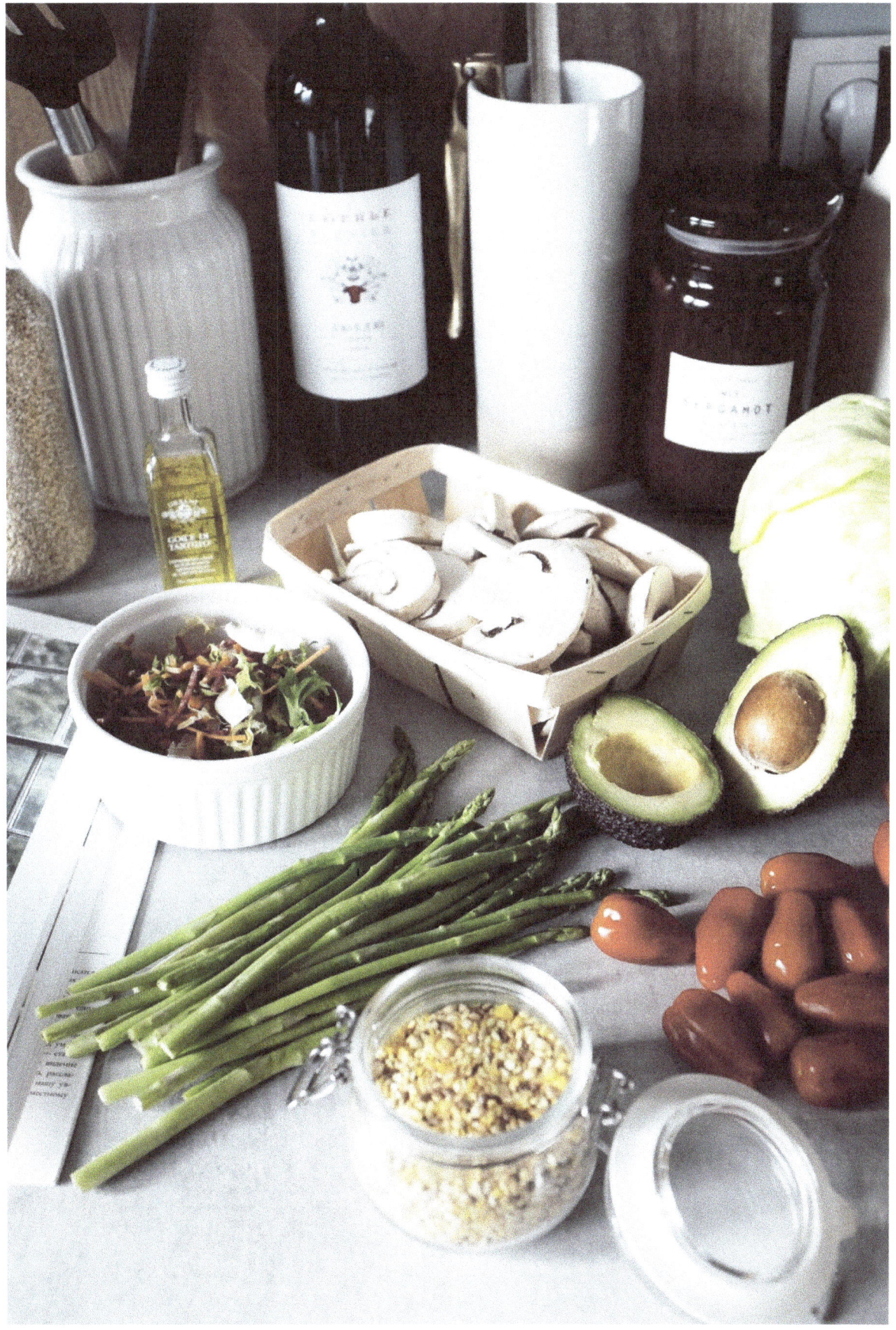

Chapter 4: Exercise

Mediterranean diet is extremely flexible, and you won't have problems while being out with friends. Many recipes in the restaurants come from this particular diet so, you are good to go as long as you do not eat junk food and food that is high in sugar.

Eat slowly and chew your food better. Put your utensils down between bites because that is going to help you slow down the process of eating.

The tips above will help you a lot, but nothing will help you more in this journey than exercising. Two years ago, one scientific research that mainly focused on the Mediterranean diet revealed that this diet is extremely beneficial and gets its full potential when exercise is included. So, to keep your weight under control and to lose weight at the same time you must exercise.

Do not force yourself, start with something easy and small. Spend 30 to 60 minutes daily on that part. Walk, run, do yoga, swim, ride a bike, or simply infiltrate yourself into a regular exercise program online or in a gym near you.

Regular physical activity does not improve only your look, it also improves your strength, mood and balance.

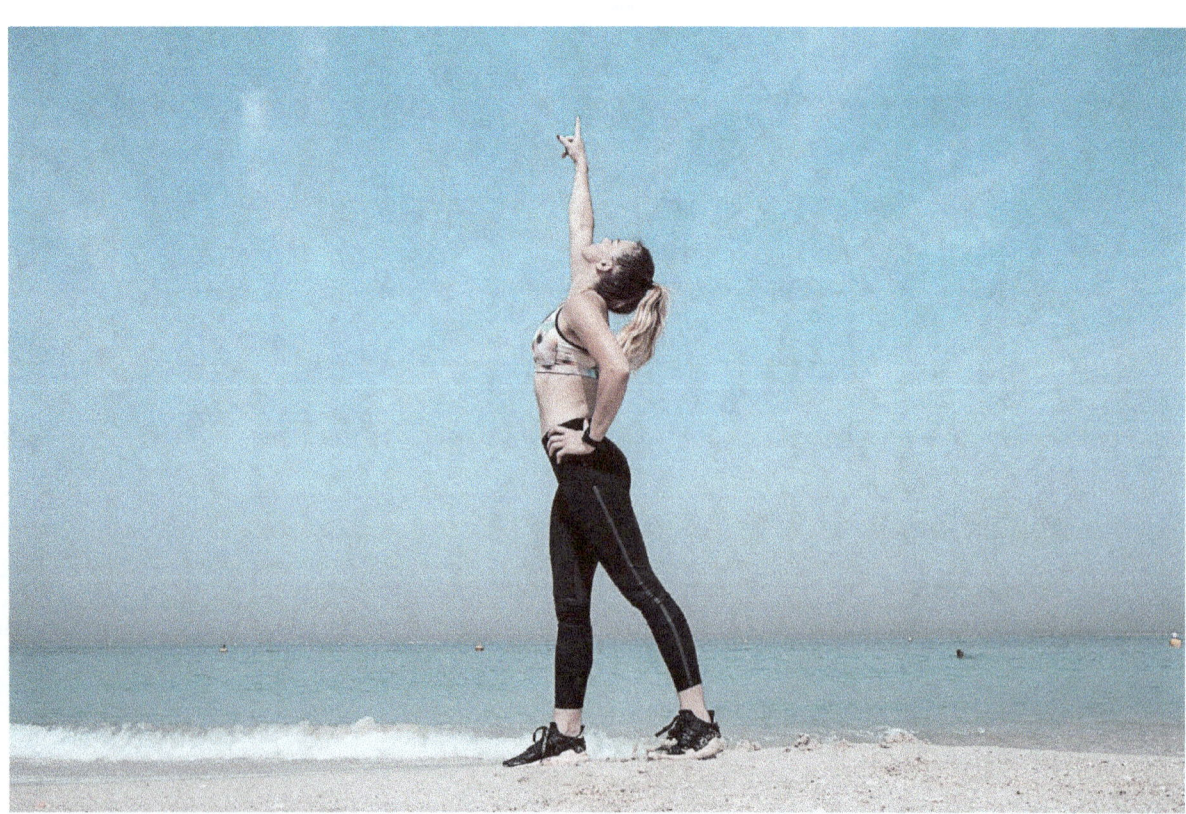

Chapter 5: The recipes in this book

This book contains 500 recipes in total. Each recipe is designed according to the rules Mediterranean diet has. Every recipe is healthy, and every recipe should be made with the best ingredients available – the organic ones. There is also a section for vegans and vegetarians. We wanted to include every person possible in this journey because this journey is all about health and improving yourself and the way you eat. At the bottom of this book you will find a meal plan that we think is going to help you a lot in the few first months. The start won't be that hard, but it is going to be challenging I must admit.

The cooking skills

It is important to know that the Mediterranean do not require hours and hours in the kitchen. The way these recipes are prepared is easy and convenient.

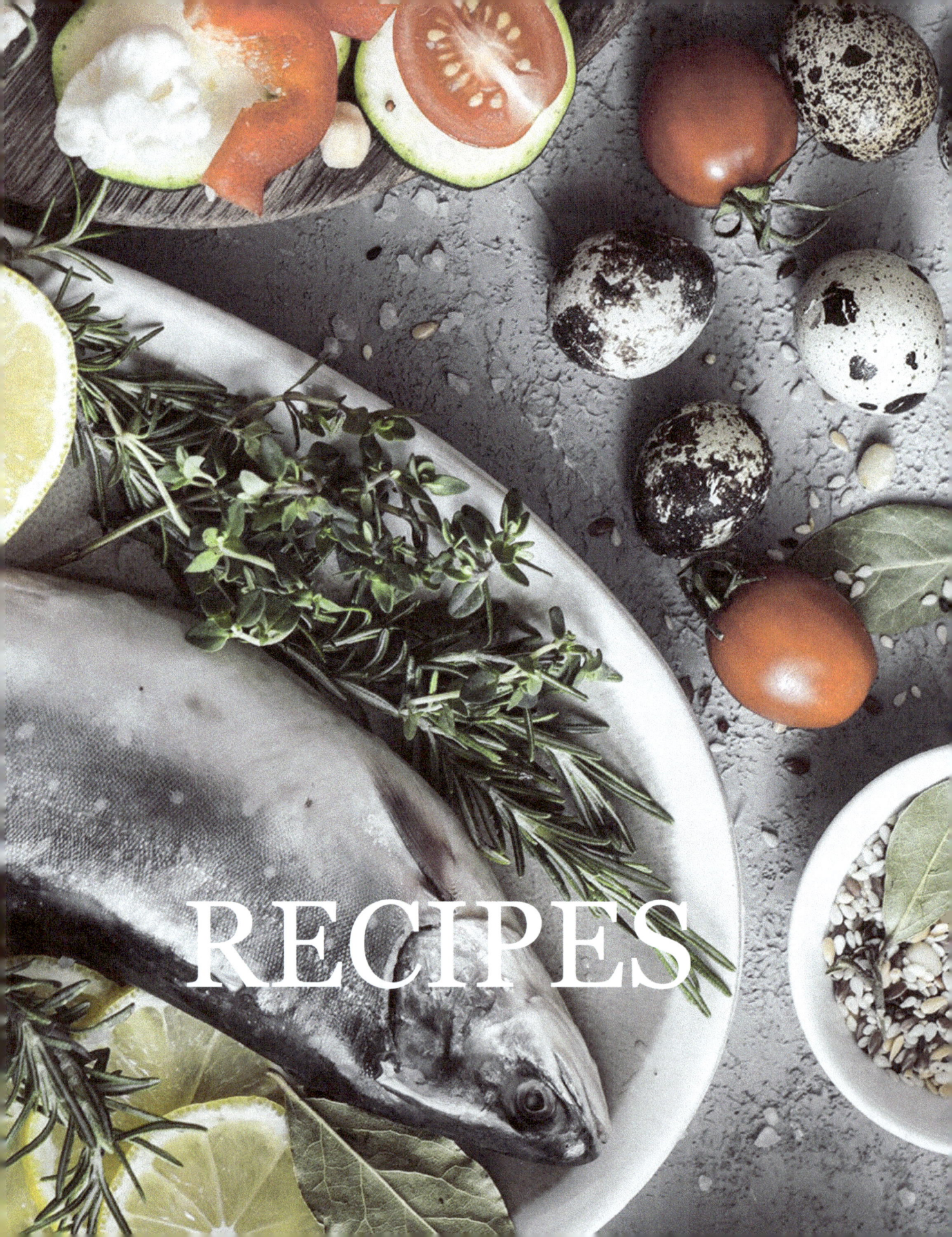

RECIPES

Pasta

Simple Mac and Cheese Pasta

COOKING: 40 MIN   SERVES: 4

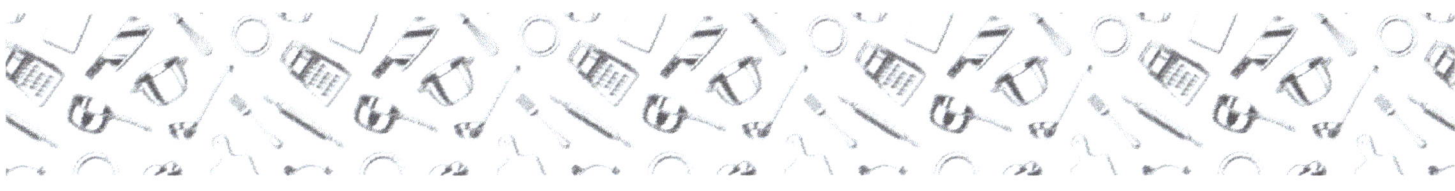

INGREDIENTS

1/2 (16 ounce) package fusilli (spiral) pasta
1/4 cup olive oil
1 tablespoon minced onion
1/4 cup all-purpose flour
2 cups milk
4 ounces processed cheese food
1/4 cup blue cheese crumbles
1/4 cup cubed Cheddar cheese
1 teaspoon salt
1 pinch ground black pepper
1/4 teaspoon dry mustard

Nutritional Value: 369 calories per serving

DIRECTIONS

Fill a large pot with lightly salted water and bring to a rolling boil over high heat. Once the water is boiling, stir in the fusilli, and return to a boil. Cook the pasta uncovered, stirring occasionally, until the pasta has cooked through, but is still firm to the bite, about 12 minutes. Drain well in a colander set in the sink.

2. Preheat oven to 400 degrees F (200 degrees C). Lightly grease a casserole dish.
3. Melt the olive oil in a large saucepan over medium heat; cook the onion in the melted olive oil until translucent, about 5 minutes.
4. Whisk the flour into the onion mixture; cook 1 minute more. Slowly pour the milk into the mixture while whisking until the milk is entirely incorporated. Add the cheese food, blue cheese, Cheddar cheese, salt, pepper, and mustard; cook and stir continually the cheese has melted and the mixture is thick; fold the pasta into the mixture. Pour the mixture into the prepared casserole dish.
5. Bake in the preheated oven until the top begins to brown, about 20 minutes.

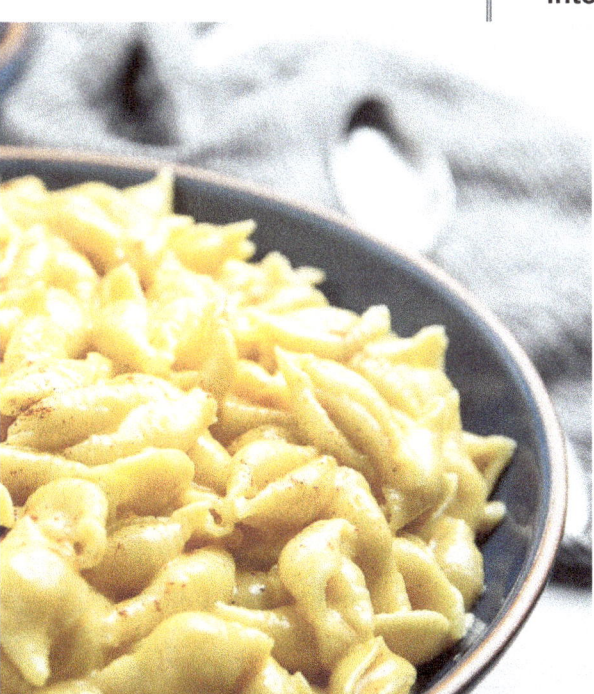

Pasta

Cold Spaghetti

COOKING: 20 MIN   SERVES: 2

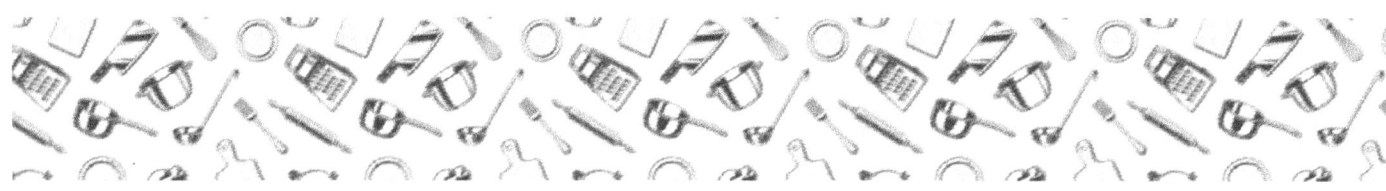

INGREDIENTS

4 ripe tomatoes - peeled and seeded
3 cloves garlic, peeled
1/3 cup chopped fresh basil
1 teaspoon olive oil
1/2 teaspoon white raw honey
1 (8 ounce) package uncooked spaghetti
1/2 cup shredded Parmesan cheese

Nutritional Value: 410 calories per serving

DIRECTIONS

1. In a blender or food processor, Mix tomatoes, garlic, basil, oil and raw honey and process until smooth. Cover and refrigerate sauce.
2. Bring a large pot of lightly salted water to a boil. Add pasta and cook for 8 to 10 minutes or until al dente; drain.
3. Remove sauce from refrigerator and pour over spaghetti. Toss to coat and serve topped with Parmesan cheese.

Pasta

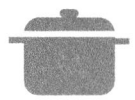 The Most Mediterranean Pasta Sauce

COOKING: 10 MIN SERVES: 2

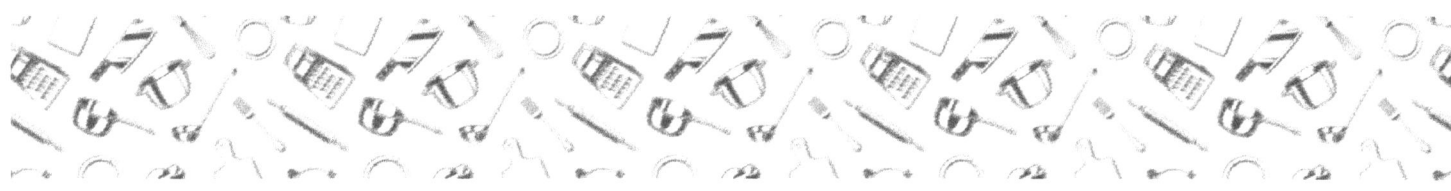

INGREDIENTS

12 ounces dry fettuccine pasta
1-pound lean ground beef (optional)
1 cup chopped onion
1 cup red bell pepper, chopped
1 tablespoon butter
1 (29 ounce) can diced tomatoes
(4 ounce) can sliced mushrooms
3 tablespoons chopped black olives
teaspoons dried oregano
1 cup shredded Cheddar cheese
1 cup shredded mozzarella cheese
1 (10.75 ounce) can condensed cream of mushroom soup
1/4 cup beef broth
1/4 cup grated Parmesan cheese

Nutritional Value: 471 calories per serving

DIRECTIONS

1. In a large skillet, heat the oil on high and add the garlic. Reduce to medium high and cook until the garlic begins to turn golden, then add the peppers. Cook until the peppers are soft and turning brown around the edges. Add the olives and crushed red pepper and stir. Pour in the wine and cook for 2 minutes.
2. Add the tomato-vegetable juice cocktail, basil, oregano, raw honey, salt and pepper. Bring to a boil and reduce heat to medium. Cook until liquid is halved. Stir in parsley. Serve over your favorite pasta.

Pasta

Carbonara Spaghetti

COOKING: 25 MIN

SERVES: 2

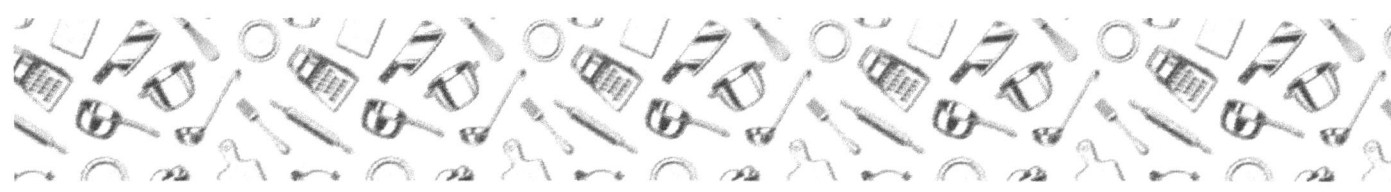

INGREDIENTS

8 oz. spaghetti
4 oz. bacon
1 green pepper
5 tbsp. Parmesan cheese
5 tbsp. chopped parsley
1-1/4 cups cream
1/4 cup butter
8 slices cooked ham, lean
1 tsp. dried oregano
1 tsp. dried basil

Nutritional Value: 471 calories per serving

DIRECTIONS

1. Cook spaghetti in boiling saltwater for 15 minutes.
2. Meanwhile, chop bacon. Core pepper and chop finely. Put bacon insaucepan, cook until crisp. Stir in cheese, parsley, cream, green pepper. Cook slowly 5 minutes.
3. Drain spaghetti, toss with butter, place in greased oven dish.
4. Roll up ham slices, lay on spaghetti, cover with bacon sauce.
5. Sprinkle with herbs. Bake at 425 degrees for 10 minutes. Serve hot.

Pasta

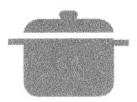

Penne with Asparagus and Shrimp

COOKING: 25 MIN

SERVES: 2

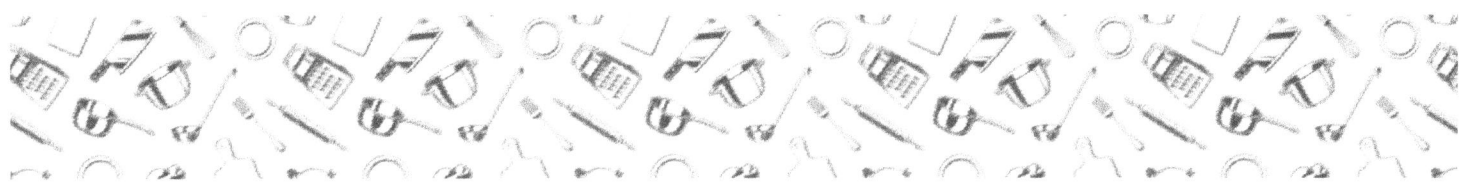

INGREDIENTS

1 cup penne pasta
2 tablespoons olive oil
2 cloves garlic, minced
1/4 cup onion, chopped
1/2 cup white wine
1/4 teaspoon crushed red pepper flakes
1 tablespoon butter
10 spears asparagus, cut into 1-inch pieces
18 peeled and deveined large shrimp
1 tablespoon lemon juice salt and pepper to taste
2 tablespoons chopped fresh flat-leaf parsley
1/4 cup grated Parmesan cheese

Nutritional Value: 471 calories per serving

DIRECTIONS

1. Bring a large pot of lightly salted water to a boil. Add penne and cook until al dente, 8 to 10 minutes; drain.
2. Meanwhile, heat the olive oil in a large skillet over medium heat. Stir in the garlic and onion and cook until the onion has softened and turned translucent, about 5 minutes. Pour in the white wine, and simmer for 2 minutes. Stir in the red pepper flakes, butter, and asparagus; cook until the asparagus is just tender, about 3 minutes. Add the shrimp and lemon juice, continue cooking until the shrimp have turned pink and are no longer translucent in the center.
3. Season to taste with salt and pepper.
4. Toss the cooked penne pasta with the shrimp and asparagus mixture. Sprinkle with parsley and Parmesan cheese to garnish.

Pasta

Fettucine Lasagna

COOKING: 25 MIN

SERVES: 2

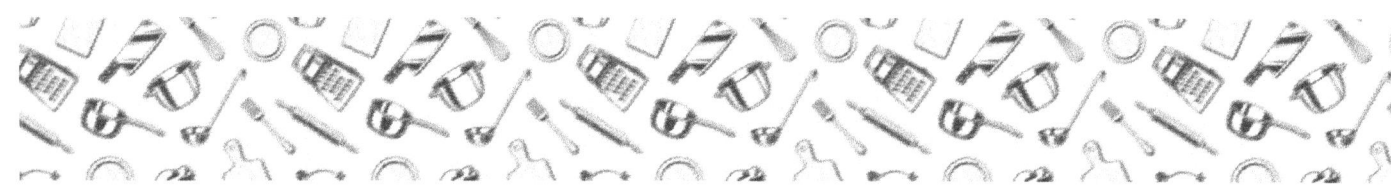

INGREDIENTS

12 ounces dry fettuccine pasta
1-pound lean ground beef (optional)
1 cup chopped onion
1 cup red bell pepper, chopped
1 tablespoon butter
1 (29 ounce) can diced tomatoes
(4 ounce) can sliced mushrooms
3 tablespoons chopped black olives
teaspoons dried oregano
1 cup shredded Cheddar cheese
1 cup shredded mozzarella cheese
1 (10.75 ounce) can condensed cream of mushroom soup
1/4 cup beef broth
1/4 cup grated Parmesan cheese

Nutritional Value: 471 calories per serving

DIRECTIONS

1. Bring a large pot of lightly salted water to a boil. Cook pasta for 8 to 10 minutes, or until al dente; drain.
2. In a large skillet, brown beef over medium heat. Drain fat from pan, and transfer meat to a bowl. In the same skillet, cook onion and bell pepper in butter until tender. Stir in tomatoes, mushrooms, olives, and beef, and season with oregano. Simmer for 10 minutes.
3. Preheat oven to 350 degrees F (175 degrees C). Lightly grease a 9x13 inch baking dish.
4. Arrange half of the cooked fettuccine in the prepared dish, top with half of the beef and vegetable mixture, and sprinkle with 1/2 cup of Cheddar cheese and 1/2 cup of mozzarella cheese. Repeat layers. Mix together soup and beef broth until smooth and pour over casserole. Sprinkle with Parmesan cheese.
5. Bake in preheated oven for 30 to 35 minutes, or until heated through

Pasta

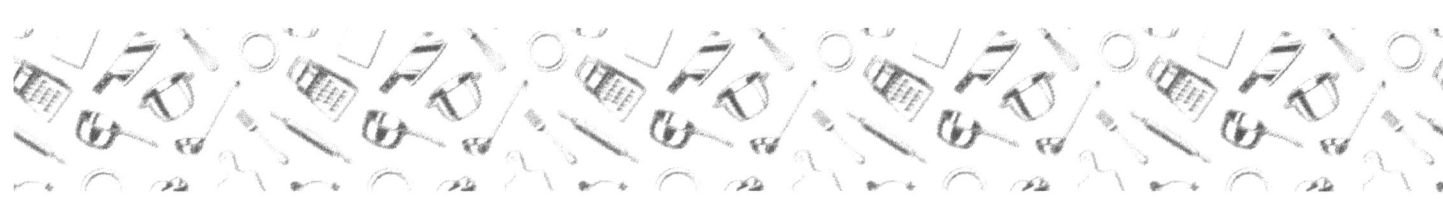

Pasta with Lentil Soup

COOKING: 25 MIN   SERVES: 2

INGREDIENTS

16 ounce) package uncooked spaghetti
(19 ounce) cans lentil soup freshly ground black pepper to taste

Nutritional Value: 410 calories per serving

DIRECTIONS

1. Bring a large pot of lightly salted water to a boil. Add spaghetti and cook for 8 to 10 minutes or until al dente; drain, but do not rinse, and return to pot. Stir in lentil soup and season with black pepper. Heat through and serve.

Pasta

Penne Key West

COOKING: 25 MIN   SERVES: 2

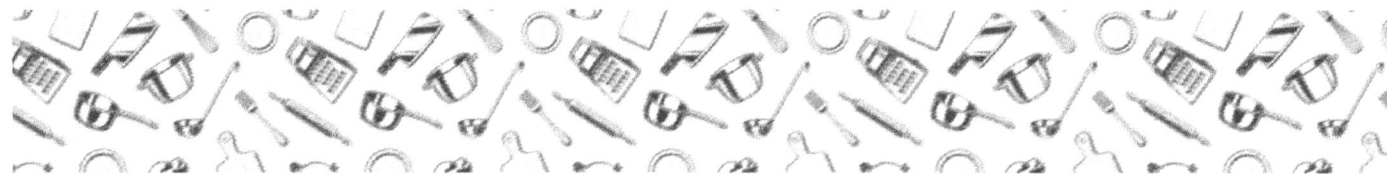

INGREDIENTS

1 (16 ounce) package penne pasta
1-pound shrimp
1-pound scallops
1 (12 ounce) jar marinated artichoke hearts, drained
1 (8 ounce) jar sun-dried tomatoes, packed in oil
1-pint heavy cream
1 cup grated Parmesan cheese
1/2 cup pitted kalamata olives

Nutritional Value: 369 calories per serving

DIRECTIONS

1. Bring a large pot of lightly salted water to a boil. Add pasta and cook for 8 to 10 minutes or until al dente; drain.
2. Heat a large heavy skillet over medium heat. Combine shrimp, scallops, artichokes and sun-dried tomatoes, then cook until shrimp turn pink. Reduce heat and stir in cream and parmesan. Toss with cooked pasta, and sprinkle olives on top.

Pasta

Interesting Pasta

COOKING: 25 MIN

SERVES: 2

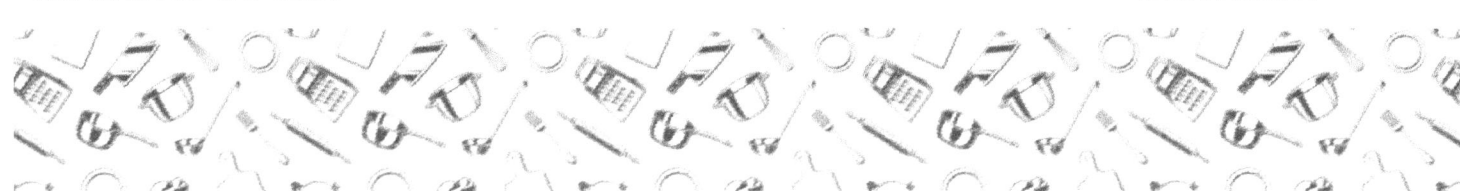

INGREDIENTS

1-pound lean ground beef
Salt
Pepper
1/2 onion
1 green bell pepper
1 (6 ounce) can tomato paste
1 tablespoon chopped garlic
1 tablespoon dried oregano
20 cherry tomatoes
1 (12 ounce) package linguine pasta

Nutritional Value: 471 calories per serving

DIRECTIONS

1. Bring a large pot of lightly salted water to a boil. Add linguine pasta and cook for 8 to 10 minutes or until al dente; drain.
2. In a large skillet over medium heat, brown the ground beef until almost cooked; about 10 minutes. Season lightly with salt and pepper.
3. Using a food processor, chop the onion finely. Wash it out and then put in the bell pepper. It should turn to liquid. That's the surprise!
4. Add tomato paste, garlic, onions, oregano, and bell pepper juice to the browned beef. Allow it to settle a little bit, folding it all together. Add the tomatoes and cover; simmer for another 15 minutes. With a fork or spatula crush the tomatoes and blend the juice into the sauce; continue simmering for about 10 more minutes. Serve over cooked pasta

Pasta

Primavera from Cali

COOKING: 25 MIN SERVES: 2

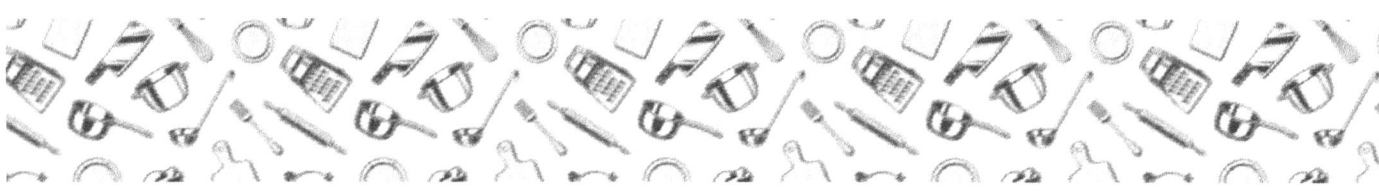

INGREDIENTS

6 ounces spaghetti
3 tablespoons olive oil 1 small onion, chopped
2 cloves garlic, minced
1 tablespoon chopped fresh basil
5 fresh mushrooms, sliced
1 (14.5 ounce) can stewed tomatoes
1 (16 ounce) package frozen mixed vegetables
1 teaspoon salt
pepper
1 tablespoon grated Parmesan cheese

Nutritional Value: 458 calories per serving

DIRECTIONS

1. In a large pot with boiling salted water cook spaghetti pasta until al dente. Drain.
2. Meanwhile, in a large skillet heat olive oil over medium heat. Add onion, garlic, basil, sliced mushrooms, and chopped tomatoes and cook for 5 minutes. Stir in California-style vegetables, salt, and ground black pepper. Cook for approximately 10 minutes, stirring often, until vegetables are tender and crisp.
3. Pour vegetable mixture over cooked and drained pasta. Toss well. Sprinkle with grated Parmesan cheese and serve.

Pasta

Macaroni and Cheese vol.2

COOKING: 25 MIN   SERVES: 2

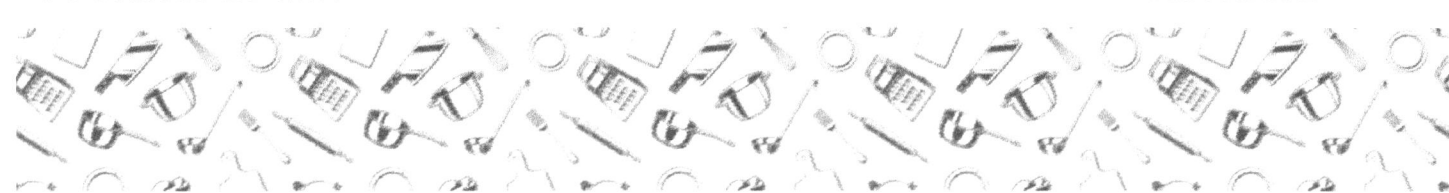

INGREDIENTS

1 (16 ounce) package elbow macaroni
1/2 cup evaporated milk
2 eggs
1 (8 ounce) container sour cream
1 teaspoon seasoning salt
1/2 teaspoon black pepper
1 1/2 cups shredded Cheddar cheese
1/2 cup grated Parmesan cheese
1 tablespoon butter

Nutritional Value: 400 calories per serving

DIRECTIONS

1. Preheat oven to 350 degrees F (175 degrees C).
2. Bring a large pot of lightly salted water to a boil. Add pasta and cook for 8 to 10 minutes or until al dente; drain and rinse with cold water.
3. In a bowl mix milk, eggs, sour cream, seasoning salt, and pepper. Layer macaroni, cheddar cheese, and milk mixture until pan is full. Sprinkle Parmesan cheese and pour melted butter on top.
4. Bake in a preheated oven for 20 to 30 minutes or until milk mixture is done.

Pasta

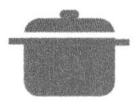 **Chicken and Tomato Pasta**

COOKING: 25 MIN   SERVES: 2

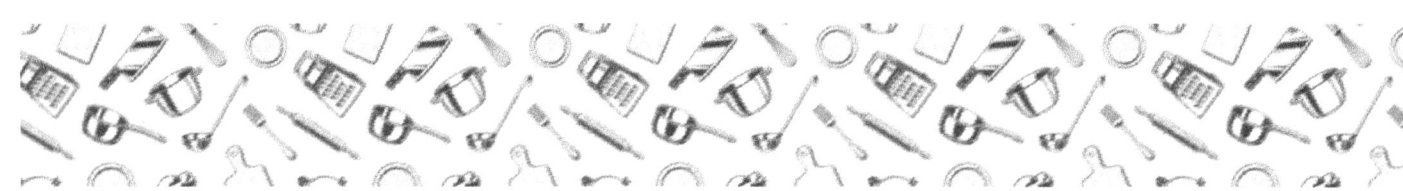

INGREDIENTS

1/2 (16 ounce) package angel hair pasta
olive oil
2 skinless, boneless chicken breast halves - chopped
2 teaspoons garlic and herb seasoning blend
1 (6 ounce) can sliced black olives, drained
(8 ounce) can sliced mushrooms, drained
(16 ounce) cans diced tomatoes
freshly grated Parmesan cheese

Nutritional Value: 250 calories per serving

DIRECTIONS

1. Bring a large pot of lightly salted water to a boil. Boil pasta for 8 to 10 minutes, or until al dente. Drain.
2. Heat olive oil in a large skillet over medium high heat. Sprinkle chicken with seasoned salt and cook for 2 to 3 minutes. Stir in drained black olives and mushrooms. Continue cooking, stirring occasionally, until chicken is golden brown. Strain chicken juices from pan and reduce heat to low. Stir in tomatoes, cover, and simmer for 15 minutes
3. Toss the pasta and chicken mixture together, sprinkle with Parmesan cheese, and serve.

Pasta

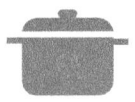 **Pasta Bake with Vegetables and Cheese**

COOKING: 25 MIN   SERVES: 2

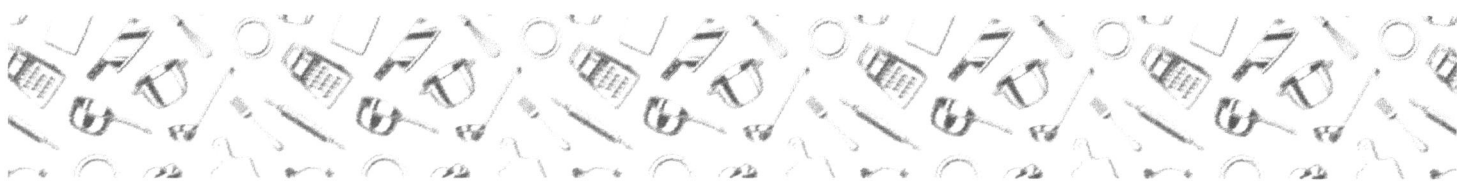

INGREDIENTS

2 tablespoons butter or olive oil
2 cloves garlic, minced
1 1/2 tablespoons flour
(12 fluid ounce) can evaporated skim milk
3/4 teaspoon salt
1/2 teaspoon hot pepper sauce (optional)
2 cups cheddar cheese
1 (16 ounce) package frozen mixed vegetables (cauliflower, red bell peppers, broccoli), thawed
3 cups bow tie or penne pasta, cooked and drained

Nutritional Value: 456 calories per serving

DIRECTIONS

1. Melt butter in large saucepan over medium heat. Add garlic; cook 2 minutes. Add flour; cook and stir 1 minute. Add milk, salt and pepper sauce. Heat to a boil, stirring constantly. Remove from heat; stir in 1 cup cheese until melted.
2. Add sauce and vegetables to pasta; toss well. Transfer to a greased medium baking dish or oval casserole. Cover with foil; bake in preheated 375 degrees F oven 15 minutes or until hot. Uncover and sprinkle with remaining cheese; bake 2 minutes more or until cheese is melted

Pasta

The Easiest Pasta on Earth

COOKING: 25 MIN   SERVES: 2

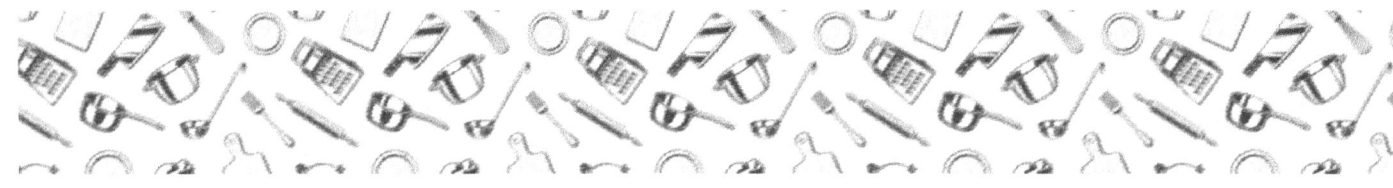

INGREDIENTS

2 cups chicken broth 2 cups heavy cream
8 ounces linguine pasta 6 slices bacon
2 cups chopped cooked chicken 1 cup frozen English peas, thawed 1 cup freshly grated Parmesan cheese

Nutritional Value: 124 calories per serving

DIRECTIONS

1. Bring chicken broth and cream to a boil in a heavy saucepan over high heat. Reduce heat to medium-low and simmer until reduced by half, about 30 minutes.
2. Bring a large pot of lightly salted water to a boil. Add linguine and cook 8 to 10 minutes or until al dente; drain and set aside in a large serving bowl.
3. Meanwhile, place bacon in a large, deep skillet. Cook over medium high heat until evenly brown. Drain, crumble and set aside.
4. Once the cream has reduced, stir in crumbled bacon, chicken, peas, and Parmesan cheese; cook for a few minutes until hot. Pour sauce over pasta to serve.

Pasta

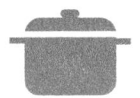

Shrimp Pasta with Feta Cheese

COOKING: 25 MIN   SERVES: 2

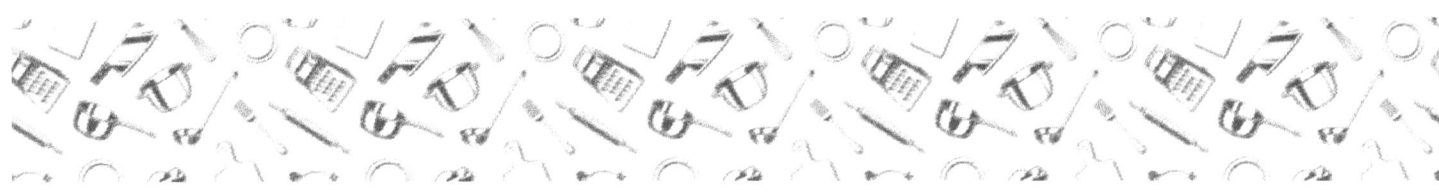

INGREDIENTS

(16 ounce) package uncooked angel hair pasta
tablespoons butter
2 tablespoons diced onion
4 ounces crumbled feta cheese
1/2-pound medium shrimp - peeled and deveined

Nutritional Value: 582 calories per serving

DIRECTIONS

1. Bring a large pot of lightly salted water to a boil. Place pasta in the pot, cook 4 minutes, until al dente, and drain. Transfer to a large bowl.
2. Melt the butter in a skillet over medium heat. Place onion in the skillet and cook until tender. Stir in shrimp, and cook 3 minutes, or until opaque. Mix in feta cheese and continue cooking 1 minute. Toss with the pasta and serve.

Pasta

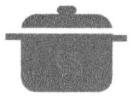

Spaghetti Casserole

COOKING: 25 MIN SERVES: 2

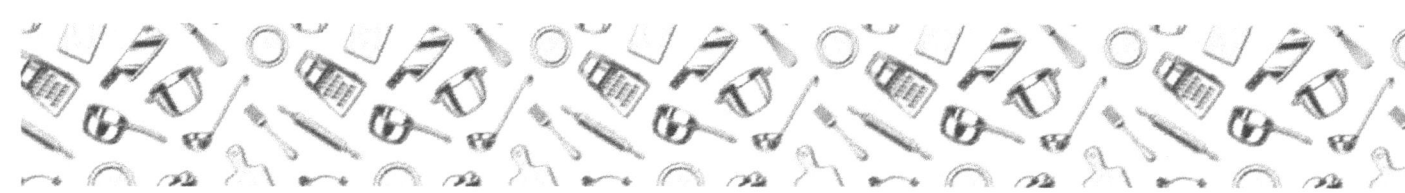

INGREDIENTS

(16 ounce) package spaghetti 2 pounds ground beef
1/4 cup chopped onion
(26.5 ounce) cans meatless spaghetti sauce
(16 ounce) container fat-free sour cream
cups shredded mozzarella cheese, divided
1/2 cup Parmesan cheese salt and black pepper to taste

Nutritional Value: 469 calories per serving

DIRECTIONS

1. Preheat oven to 350 degrees F (175 degrees C). Grease a deep 9x13 inch baking dish.
2. Bring a large pot of salted water to a boil over high heat. Stir in the spaghetti. Boil the pasta until cooked through but still firm to the bite, 8 to 10 minutes. Drain well.
3. Brown ground beef and onion in a large skillet over high heat; drain fat. Stir in the spaghetti sauce, sour cream, and 1 cup of the mozzarella. Mix in the cooked pasta. Transfer pasta mixture to prepared baking dish. Top with remaining 1 cup of mozzarella and the Parmesan cheese. Cover pan with aluminum foil.
4. Bake in preheated oven until hot and bubbly, about 30 minutes.

Pasta

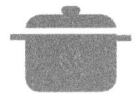

Pumpkin Pasta

COOKING: 25 MIN

SERVES: 2

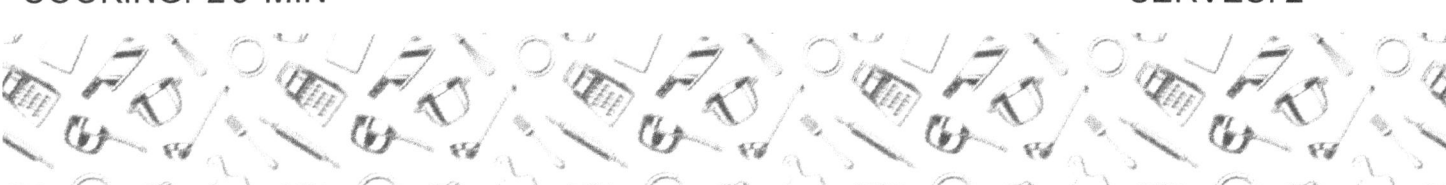

INGREDIENTS

10 ounces dry fettuccini noodles
1 tablespoon olive oil
pound peeled, seeded and grated pumpkin
1/2 tablespoons tomato paste
4 tablespoons lite sour cream
1 teaspoon chili powder

Nutritional Value: 452 calories per serving

DIRECTIONS

1. Bring a large pot of lightly salted water to a boil. Add pasta and cook for 8 to 10 minutes or until al dente; drain and reserve.
2. In a large skillet over medium heat, warm oil and cook pumpkin for about 10 minutes or until it begins to break apart.
3. Add tomato paste, sour cream and chili powder to taste; mix well. The mixture should be mushy and an even golden-orange color.
4. Scoop spoonfuls of the pumpkin mixture over the pasta; mix well to coat and serve.

Pasta

Spaghetti Chicken

COOKING: 25 MIN   SERVES: 2

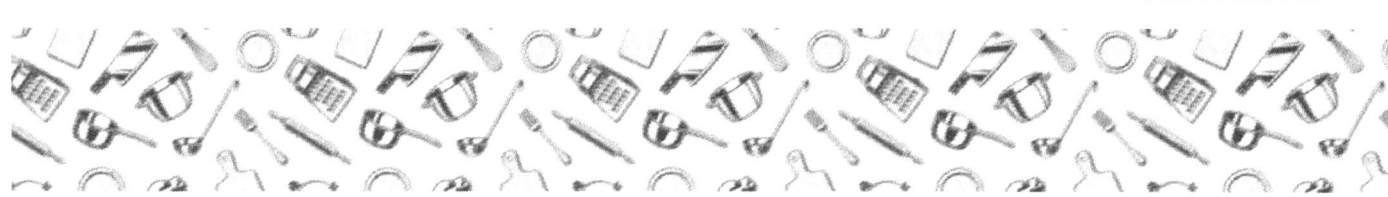

INGREDIENTS

1-pound spaghetti
1-pound boneless chicken breast halves, cooked and chopped
1 (10.75 ounce) can condensed cream of mushroom soup
1 (4.5 ounce) can sliced mushrooms
1 onion, chopped
4 cups frozen cauliflower and carrots
1 (10 ounce) can diced tomatoes with green chili peppers (optional)
1-pound cubed processed cheese food

Nutritional Value: 326 calories per serving

DIRECTIONS

1. Cook pasta in a large pot of boiling, salted water until al dente.
2. In a large bowl, mix together cooked spaghetti, chopped chicken, cream of mushroom soup, canned mushrooms, onion, and vegetables. Mix in tomatoes with chilies, if desired. Pour mixture into a greased 2-quart casserole dish. Place cubed processed cheese food on top of dish.
3. Bake in a preheated 350-degree F (175 degrees C) for 30 minutes, or until cheese is bubbly and melted.

Pasta

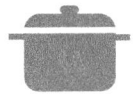

Pesto Pasta with Mint

COOKING: 25 MIN   SERVES: 2

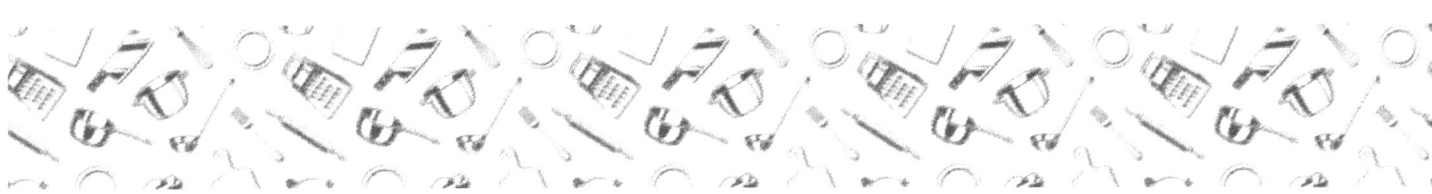

INGREDIENTS

1 (16 ounce) package uncooked linguini pasta
6 tomatoes, seeded and chopped
20 fresh basil leaves
10 fresh mint leaves
cloves garlic, chopped
1/2 cup pine nuts
tablespoons Parmesan cheese
2 tablespoons ricotta cheese
1 1/2 tablespoons olive oil salt and pepper to taste

Nutritional Value: 236 calories per serving

DIRECTIONS

1. Bring a large pot of lightly salted water to a boil. Place linguini in the pot, and cook for 8 to 10 minutes, until al dente. Drain, reserving 1 1/2 tablespoons water.
2. In a blender or food processor, blend the reserved water, tomatoes, basil, mint, garlic, pine nuts, Parmesan cheese, ricotta cheese, olive oil, salt, and pepper until smooth. Toss with the cooked pasta to serve.

Pasta

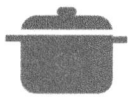

Pasta Bake vol.2

COOKING: 25 MIN

SERVES: 2

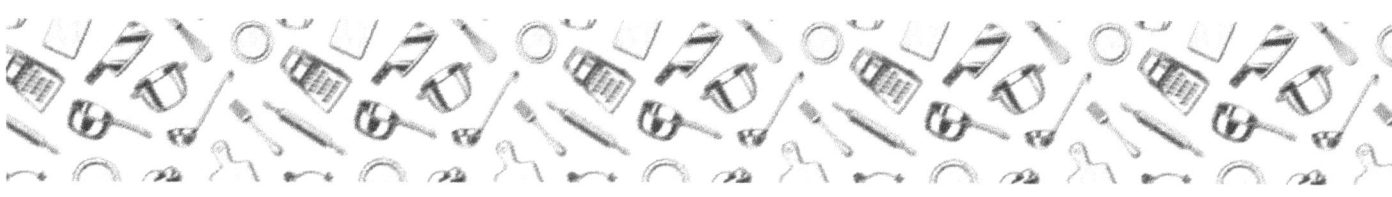

INGREDIENTS

8 ounces Mostaccioli pasta
1-pound lean ground beef
1 onion, chopped
1 (4 ounce) can mushrooms, drained
1 (28 ounce) jar spaghetti sauce
2 cups shredded mozzarella cheese

Nutritional Value: 455 calories per serving

DIRECTIONS

1. Bring a large pot of lightly salted boil water to a boil. Cook Mostaccioli pasta in boiling water for 8 to 10 minutes, or until al dente. Drain well.
2. Meanwhile, cook ground beef and chopped onions in a skillet over medium heat until browned.
3. In a large bowl, mix together the mushrooms, spaghetti sauce, shredded mozzarella cheese, pasta, and browned ground beef and onion mixture. Transfer to a greased, 9x13 inch casserole dish
4. Bake at 325 degrees F (165 degrees C) for 20 minutes, or until very hot.

Pasta

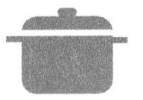 Ham and Pea Spaghetti

COOKING: 25 MIN   SERVES: 2

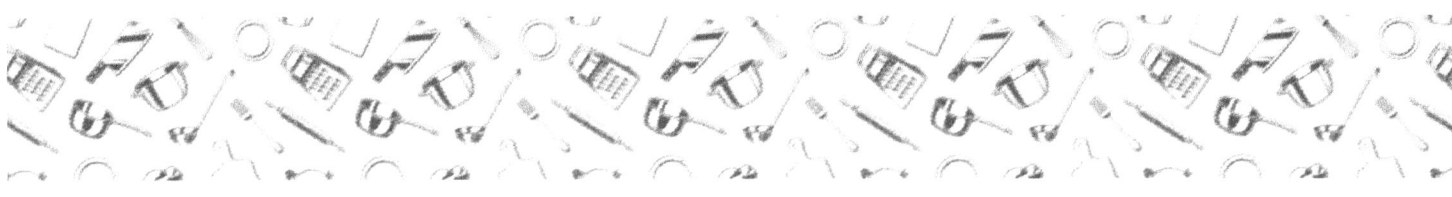

INGREDIENTS

1 8 oz. package spaghetti
1/4 cup butter
1 tbsp. flour
1/4 tsp. salt
1/4 tsp. cracked pepper
1-1/2 cups half & half
1 10 oz. package frozen peas, thawed
1 cup fontina cheese
1 cup mozzarella cheese
1 4 oz. package sliced, cooked ham

Nutritional Value: 369 calories per serving

DIRECTIONS

1. Prepare spaghetti as label directs. Drain, keep warm.
2. Meanwhile, in 3-quart saucepan, over low heat, melt butter; stir in flour, salt, pepper; gradually stir in half and half. Cook, stirring, until thickened. Add peas (thawed) and shredded cheeses, stir in ham, heat.
3. In large bowl, toss spaghetti and cheese mixture until spaghetti is well coated. Serve immediately.

Pasta

 **Tuscan Style Pasta**

COOKING: 25 MIN   SERVES: 2

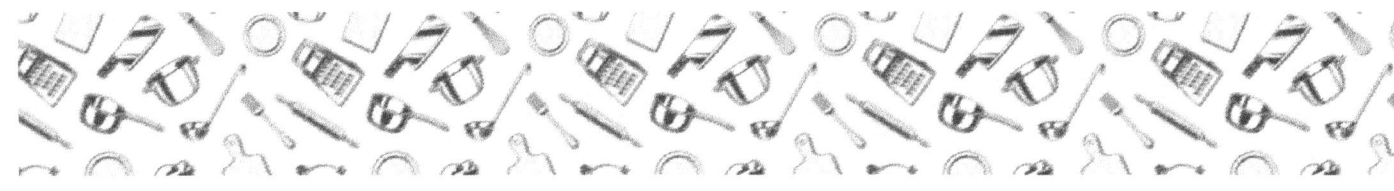

INGREDIENTS

1-pound ziti or penne pasta
1/4 cup extra-virgin olive oil
5 large garlic cloves, finely chopped
1/4-pound curly escarole, sliced
1 (16 ounce) can cannellini beans, drained and rinsed
1 (14.5 ounce) can diced tomatoes with juice, undrained
2/3 cup dry white wine or canned vegetable broth
Salt and freshly ground pepper, to taste
1/4 cup fresh basil leaves, thinly sliced

Nutritional Value: 456 calories per serving

DIRECTIONS

1. Cook pasta according to the package Instructions.
2. Heat oil in a large skillet over medium-high heat. Add garlic and cook until slightly browned (less than a minute). Add escarole, stirring occasionally until wilted, about 2 minutes. Add beans, tomatoes with their juice and wine. Simmer 5 minutes, stirring occasionally. Season to taste with salt and pepper; stir in basil and heat through. Drain pasta and toss with the sauce.

Pasta

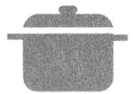

Siciliano Pasta

COOKING: 25 MIN   SERVES: 2

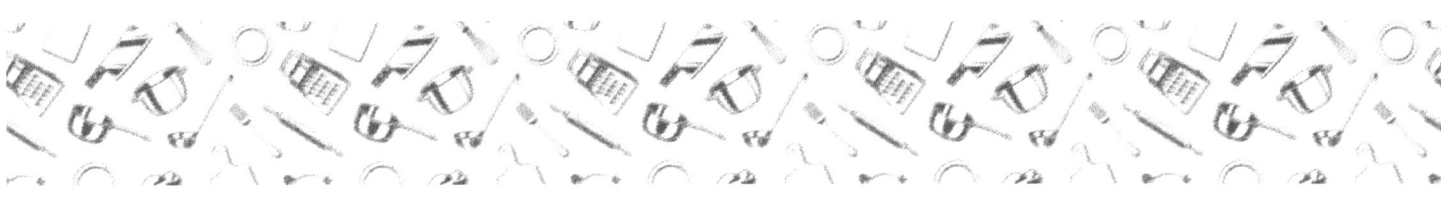

INGREDIENTS

1 (16 ounce) package uncooked farfalle pasta
1/4 cup olive oil
3 cloves chopped garlic
1 teaspoon crushed red pepper flakes
2 tablespoons lemon juice
1/2 cup pine nuts
1 (2.25 ounce) can sliced black olives
1/2 cup chopped sun-dried tomatoes
1 cup crumbled feta cheese salt and pepper to taste

Nutritional Value: 478 calories per serving

DIRECTIONS

1. Bring a large pot of lightly salted water to a boil. Place farfalle pasta in the pot, cook for 8 to 10 minutes, until al dente, and drain.
2. Heat the oil in a large skillet over medium heat and cook the garlic until lightly browned. Mix in red pepper and lemon juice. Stir in the pine nuts, olives, and sun-dried tomatoes. Toss in the cooked pasta and feta cheese. Season with salt and pepper

Pasta

Pomodoro Pasta

COOKING: 25 MIN SERVES: 2

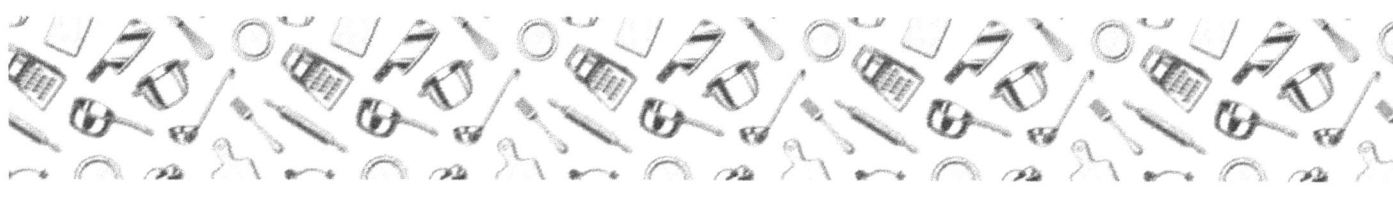

INGREDIENTS

2 (8 ounce) packages angel hair pasta
1/4 cup olive oil 1/2 onion, chopped
4 cloves garlic, minced
2 cups roma (plum) tomatoes, diced
2 tablespoons balsamic vinegar
1 (10.75 ounce) can low-sodium chicken broth
1 crushed red pepper to taste
freshly ground black pepper to taste
2 tablespoons chopped fresh basil
1/4 cup grated Parmesan cheese

Nutritional Value: 452 calories per serving

DIRECTIONS

1. Bring a large pot of lightly salted water to a boil. Add pasta and cook for 8 minutes or until al dente; drain.
2. Pour olive oil in a large deep skillet over high heat. Sauté onions and garlic until lightly browned. Reduce heat to medium-high and add tomatoes, vinegar and chicken broth; simmer for about 8 minutes.
3. Stir in red pepper, black pepper, basil and cooked pasta, tossing thoroughly with sauce. Simmer for about 5 more minutes and serve topped with grated cheese.

Pasta

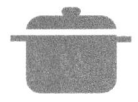

Basil and Tomato Pasta

COOKING: 25 MIN SERVES: 2

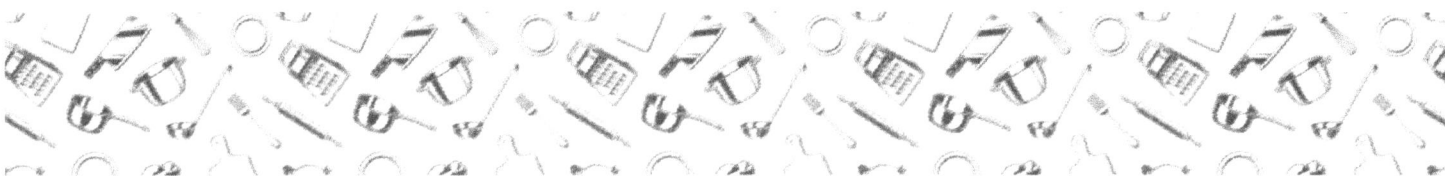

INGREDIENTS

10 ounces dry fusilli/spiral pasta
6 tablespoons olive oil
2 cloves crushed garlic
1 small onion, finely chopped
2 cups diced tomatoes
6 leaves fresh basil, torn
3 tablespoons grated Parmesan cheese
1 1/2 cups crumbled feta cheese salt and pepper to taste

Nutritional Value: 541 calories per serving

DIRECTIONS

1. Bring a large pot of lightly salted water to a boil. Add fusilli pasta and cook for 8 to 10 minutes or until al dente; drain.
2. Mix olive oil, garlic, onion, tomatoes and basil; let sit at room temperature.
3. Toss warm pasta with Parmesan and feta. Stir in tomato mixture and sprinkle on salt and pepper. You can add more Parmesan if desired. Serve immediately.

Pasta

Mac and Cheese vol.3

COOKING: 25 MIN   SERVES: 2

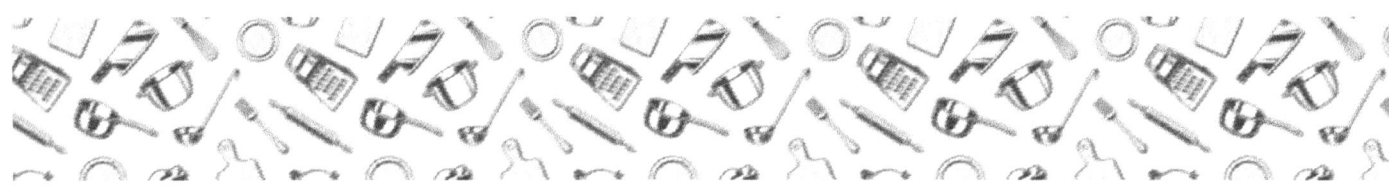

INGREDIENTS

1 (8 ounce) package elbow macaroni
1 (8 ounce) package shredded sharp Cheddar cheese
1 (12 ounce) container small curd cottage cheese
1 (8 ounce) container sour cream
1/4 cup grated Parmesan cheese
 salt and pepper to taste
1 cup dry breadcrumbs
1/4 cup butter, melted

Nutritional Value: 455 calories per serving

DIRECTIONS

1. Preheat oven to 350 degrees F (175 degrees C). Bring a large pot of lightly salted water to a boil, add pasta, and cook until done; drain.
2. In 9x13 inch baking dish, stir together macaroni, shredded Cheddar cheese, cottage cheese, sour cream, Parmesan cheese, salt and pepper. In a small bowl, mix together breadcrumbs and melted butter. Sprinkle topping over macaroni mixture.
3. Bake 30 to 35 minutes, or until top is golden.

Pasta

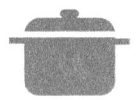

Rigatoni with Bean and Sausage

COOKING: 25 MIN   SERVES: 2

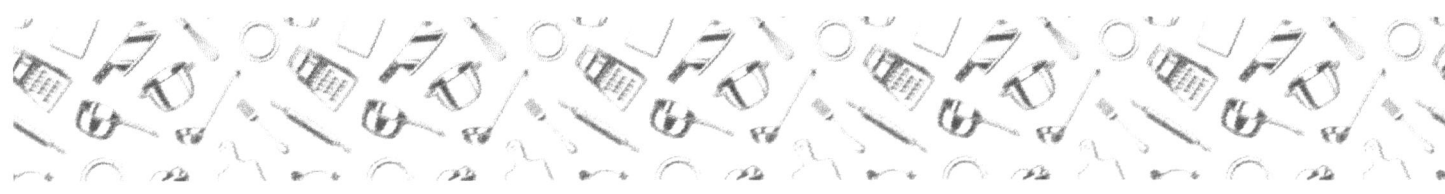

INGREDIENTS

8 ounces uncooked rigatoni or penne pasta
1 (15 ounce) can great Northern beans, rinsed and drained
1 (14.5 ounce) can stewed tomatoes
1 (10 ounce) package frozen chopped spinach, thawed and drained
1/2 pound reduced-fat smoked turkey kielbasa, halved and sliced
5 tablespoons tomato paste
1/4 cup chicken broth
1 1/2 teaspoons Italian seasoning
1/4 cup shredded Parmesan cheese

Nutritional Value: 364 calories per serving

DIRECTIONS

1. Cook pasta according to package Instructions; drain. In a bowl, Mix the pasta, beans, tomatoes, tomato paste, broth and seasoning. Transfer to a 2-qt. baking dish coated with nonstick cooking spray. Sprinkle with Parmesan cheese. Bake, uncovered, at 375 degrees F for 15-20 minutes or until heated through.

Pasta

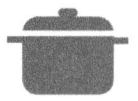 **Penne, Goat Cheese and Arugula Pasta**

COOKING: 25 MIN   SERVES: 2

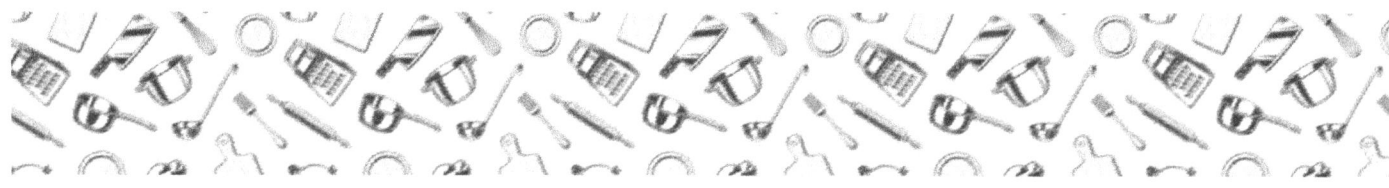

INGREDIENTS

5 1/2 ounces goat cheese
2 cups coarsely chopped arugula, stems included
cup quartered cherry tomatoes
1/4 cup olive oil
3 teaspoons minced garlic
1/2 teaspoon ground black pepper
1/2 teaspoon salt
8 ounces penne pasta

Nutritional Value: 455 calories per serving

DIRECTIONS

1. Cook pasta in a large pot of boiling salted water until al dente.
2. Crumble goat cheese into a large serving bowl. Add arugula, cherry tomatoes, olive oil, garlic, and salt and pepper.
3. Drain pasta and toss with goat cheese mixture.

Pasta

Noodles vol.2

COOKING: 25 MIN   SERVES: 2

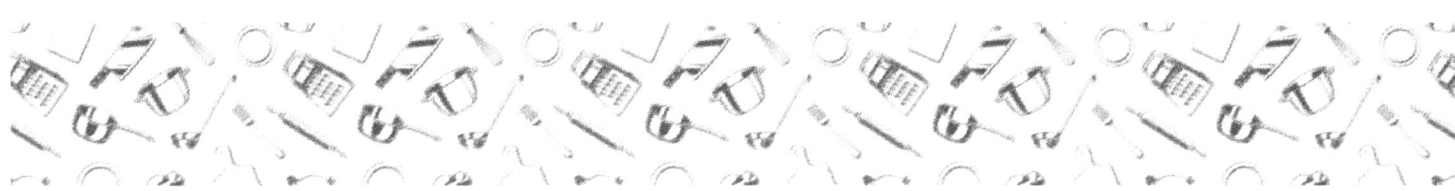

INGREDIENTS

1 (16 ounce) package uncooked linguini pasta
1 cup soy sauce
1/2 cup extra virgin olive oil
1/2 cup white raw honey
1/3 cup distilled white vinegar
1 tablespoon sesame seeds
1 (10 ounce) package mixed baby salad greens
1 (8 ounce) package imitation crabmeat, flaked
1 bunch chopped cilantro
1 avocado - peeled, pitted and diced

Nutritional Value: 321 calories per serving

DIRECTIONS

1. Bring a large pot of lightly salted water to a boil. Place linguini pasta in the pot, cook for 8 to 10 minutes, until al dente, and drain.
2. In a bowl, whisk together the soy sauce, olive oil, raw honey, vinegar, and sesame seeds.
3. In a large bowl, toss the cooked pasta with the soy sauce dressing, greens, imitation crabmeat, cilantro, and avocado. Chill until serving.

Pasta

 **Basil and Red Pepper Pasta**

COOKING: 25 MIN SERVES: 2

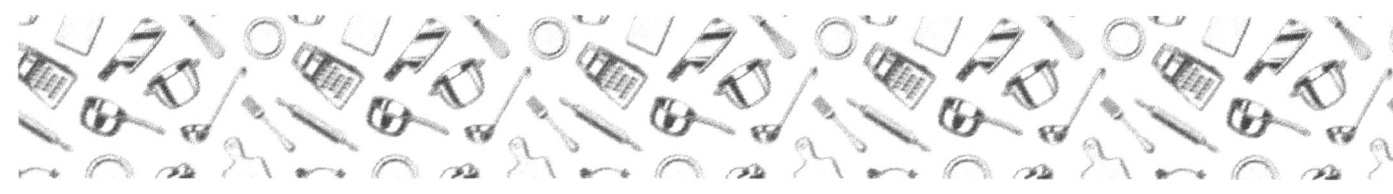

INGREDIENTS

2 cups whole wheat penne pasta, uncooked
1 (300 g) jar roasted red peppers, drained and chopped
125 grams Cream Cheese
1/2 cup skim milk
1/2 cup fresh basil leaves
2 tablespoons Kraft 100% Light Parmesan Grated Cheese
450 grams boneless skinless chicken breasts, bite-size pieces

Nutritional Value: 360 calories per serving

DIRECTIONS

1. Cook pasta as directed on package. Meanwhile, place peppers, cream cheese spread, milk, basil and Parmesan cheese in blender; cover. Blend until smooth; set aside
2. Spray large skillet with cooking spray. Add chicken; cook on medium-high heat 3 min., stirring frequently. Stir in pepper mixture. Reduce heat to medium; cook 5 min. or until heated through, stirring frequently.
3. Drain pasta. Add to chicken mixture; stir gently until well blended.

Pasta

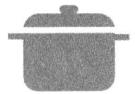

Noodles from Poland

COOKING: 25 MIN   SERVES: 2

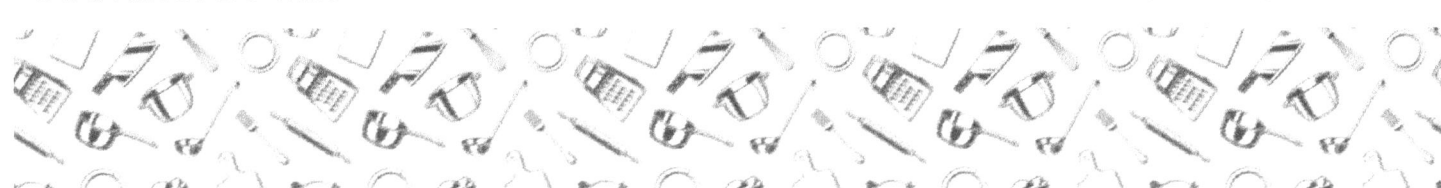

INGREDIENTS

Medium head shredded cabbage
red onions, slice into strips
1/2 cup butter
1 (16 ounce) package wide egg noodles
salt to taste
ground black pepper to taste

Nutritional Value: 547 calories per serving

DIRECTIONS

1. Cook pasta in a large pot of boiling salted water.
2. Meanwhile, heat butter or olive oil in a skillet over medium heat. Saute cabbage and onions until tender.
3. Drain pasta and return to the pot. Add cabbage and onion mixture to the noodles, and toss. Season with salt and pepper to taste.

Pasta

Taco Pasta

COOKING: 25 MIN

SERVES: 2

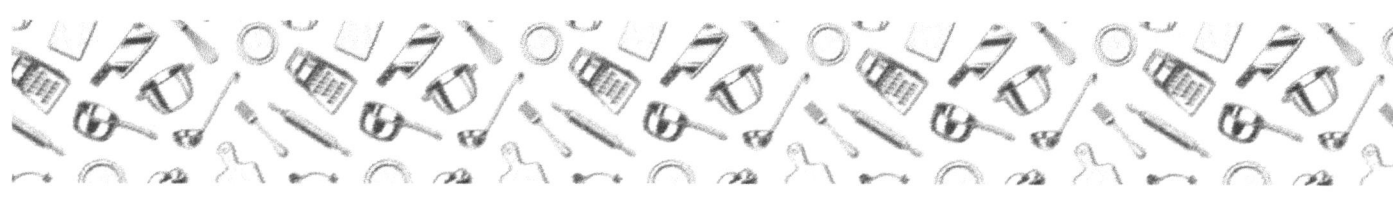

INGREDIENTS

16 ounces dry fettuccine pasta
1-pound lean ground beef
1 (1.25 ounce) package taco seasoning mix
4 ounces shredded Cheddar cheese
3 tomatoes, diced
salt to taste
ground black pepper to taste
1 pinch garlic powder
3/4 (6 ounce) can black olives, drained and chopped
2 tablespoons grated Parmesan cheese

Nutritional Value: 326 calories per serving

DIRECTIONS

1. Cook pasta in a large pot of boiling salted water until al dente. Drain.
2. Meanwhile, in a large skillet cook ground beef. Drain excess grease. Add taco seasoning packet as directed on package.
3. Transfer pasta to a large bowl. Toss with cooked meat mixture, prepared cheese, and tomatoes. If desired, add sliced olives.
4. Season to taste with salt, pepper, and garlic powder. Sprinkle with grated Parmesan cheese. Serve immediately.

Pasta

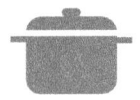 Shrimp Garlic Pasta

COOKING: 25 MIN   SERVES: 2

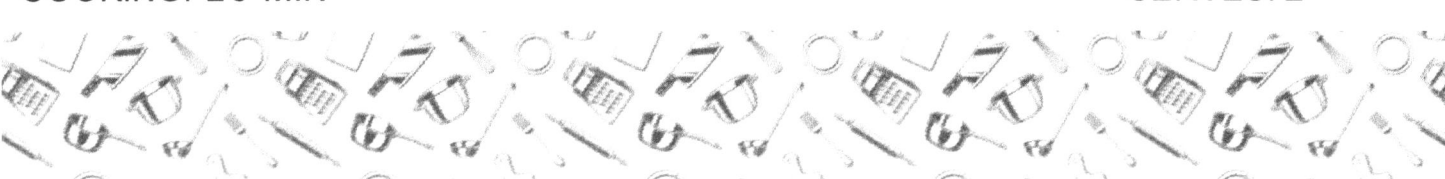

INGREDIENTS

1-pound vermicelli pasta
1 tablespoon olive oil
1-pound medium shrimp - peeled and deveined
3 tablespoons minced garlic
2 tablespoons butter
2 tablespoons grated Parmesan cheese

Nutritional Value: 411 calories per serving

DIRECTIONS

1. Cook pasta in a large pot of boiling water with olive oil until al dente.
2. Meanwhile, place the shrimp in boiling salted water for 3 to 5 minutes, just until they turn pink. Cooking time will depend on the size of the shrimp. Remove the tails, and place in a bowl of warm water.
3. In a microwave safe bowl, mix butter or olive oil and minced garlic. Microwave on high for 45 seconds, or until melted. Stir.
4. Drain pasta, and transfer to a serving dish. Toss with garlic butter and shrimp. Sprinkle with grated Parmesan cheese. Serve warm.

Pasta

 **Tequila Pasta**

COOKING: 25 MIN   SERVES: 2

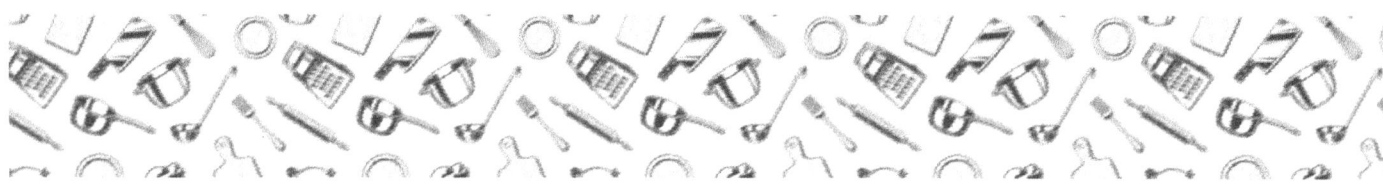

INGREDIENTS

1 tablespoon butter
1/2 onion, chopped
2 cloves garlic, thinly sliced
1/2 tablespoon chopped pickled jalapeno pepper
1 (14.4 ounce) can diced tomatoes, undrained
1 1/2 tablespoons tequila
1/4 cup water
1 (8 ounce) bottle clam juice
1 pinch crushed red pepper
1/4-pound dried elbow macaroni
1 lime, juiced

Nutritional Value: 333 calories per serving

DIRECTIONS

1. **Melt butter in a large skillet over medium heat. Stir in onion, garlic, and jalapeno; cook until onion is soft and translucent. Stir in tomatoes, tequila, water, clam juice, and red pepper. Bring to a boil, then add macaroni. Cover, and simmer, stirring frequently, until pasta is tender, about 10 minutes. Remove from heat and stir in lime juice.**

Pasta

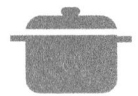

Tortellini, Steak and Caesar

COOKING: 25 MIN   SERVES: 2

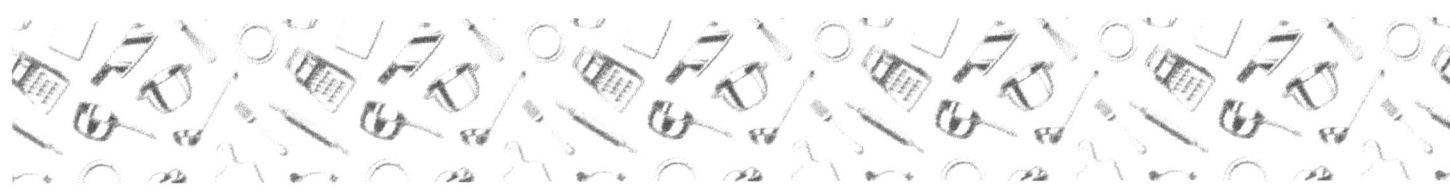

INGREDIENTS

1 (9 ounce) package cheese tortellini
1-pound flank steak garlic powder to taste salt and pepper to taste
1 tablespoon olive oil
heads romaine lettuce, torn into bite-size pieces
2 (2.25 ounce) cans small pitted black olives, drained
1 cup Caesar-style croutons
small fresh tomatoes, chopped
1 (8 ounce) bottle Caesar salad dressing

Nutritional Value: 456 calories per serving

DIRECTIONS

1. Bring a large pot of lightly salted water to a boil. Place pasta in the pot, cook for 7 to 9 minutes, until al dente, and drain.
2. Preheat the oven broiler. Season steak with garlic powder, salt, and pepper; rub with olive oil. Place steak in a baking dish, and broil 5 minutes on each side, or to desired doneness. Slice diagonally into thin strips.
3. In a bowl, toss the cooked tortellini, lettuce, olives, croutons, tomatoes, and dressing. Top with steak strips to serve.

Pasta

Ricotta Spaghetti

COOKING: 25 MIN   SERVES: 2

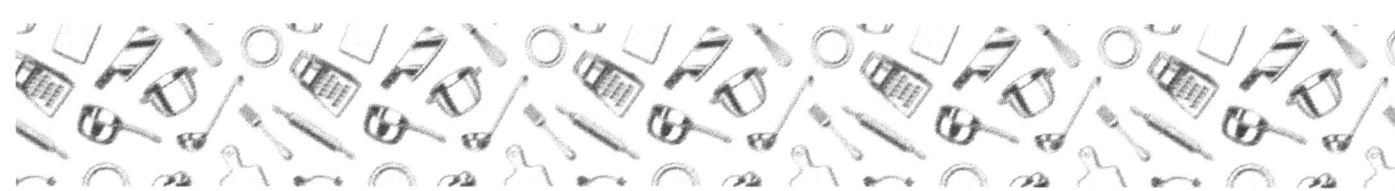

INGREDIENTS

3/4-pound spaghetti
1 clove garlic, minced
cup part-skim ricotta cheese
3 teaspoons chopped fresh basil
salt and ground black pepper to taste
2 tablespoons grated Parmesan cheese

Nutritional Value: 312 calories per serving

DIRECTIONS

1. Fill a large pot with lightly salted water and bring to a rolling boil over high heat. Once the water is boiling, stir in the spaghetti and return to a boil. Cook the pasta uncovered, stirring occasionally, until the pasta has cooked through, but is still firm to the bite, about 12 minutes. Drain well in a colander set in the sink, reserving 2 tablespoons of the cooking water.
2. Stir the garlic, ricotta, and basil in a saucepan over medium-low until hot, about 4 minutes. Season to taste with salt and pepper; stir in the spaghetti and reserved water from cooking the pasta.

Pasta

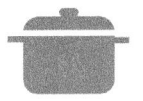

Salami and Bacon Spaghetti

COOKING: 25 MIN SERVES: 2

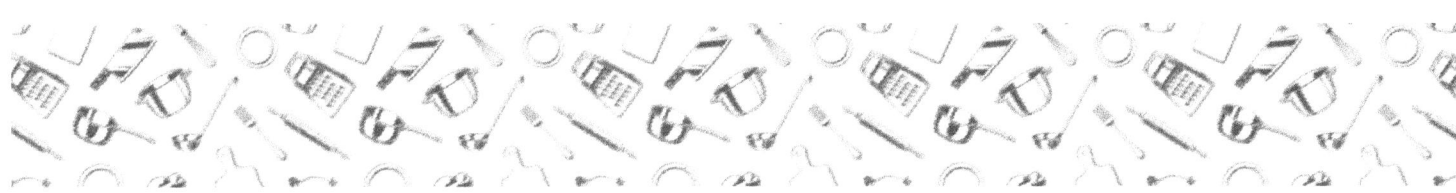

INGREDIENTS

(16 ounce) package uncooked spaghetti
3 tablespoons olive oil
1 tablespoon butter
1/4-pound hard salami, diced
2 slices bacon, chopped
1 clove garlic, chopped 1 leek, thinly sliced
salt and pepper, to taste
3 tablespoons chopped fresh basil
2 tomatoes, diced
4 tablespoons grated Parmesan cheese

Nutritional Value: 456 calories per serving

DIRECTIONS

1. Bring a large pot of lightly salted water to a boil. Cook pasta in boiling water for 8 to 10 minutes or until al dente; drain.
2. Meanwhile, heat the olive oil and butter in a large skillet over medium heat. Place salami and bacon in the skillet; cook until just starting to crisp. Stir in garlic and leek; season with salt and pepper and cook 2 minutes more. Stir in tomatoes and 1 tablespoon basil; cook 1 minute more.
3. Mix the cooked pasta into the contents of the skillet, along with 3 tablespoons Parmesan. Serve topped with remaining Parmesan and basil.

Pasta

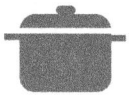 **Spinach and Feta Mostaccioli**

COOKING: 25 MIN   SERVES: 2

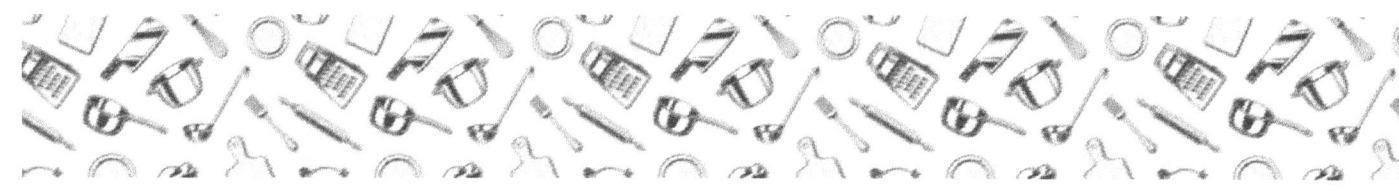

INGREDIENTS

8 ounces penne pasta
2 tablespoons olive oil
3 cups chopped tomatoes
10 ounces fresh spinach, washed and chopped
1 clove garlic, minced
8 ounces tomato basil feta cheese
salt to taste
ground black pepper to taste

Nutritional Value: 325 calories per serving

DIRECTIONS

1. Cook pasta according to package Instructions. Drain, and set aside.
2. Heat oil in a large pot. Add tomatoes, spinach, and garlic; cook and stir 2 minutes, or until spinach is wilted and mixture is thoroughly heated. Add pasta and cheese; cook 1 minute. Season to taste with salt and pepper.

Pasta

Shrimp Garlic Pasta

COOKING: 25 MIN SERVES: 2

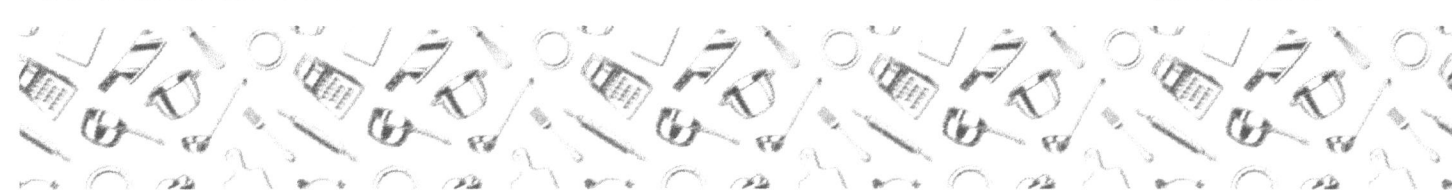

INGREDIENTS

1-pound vermicelli pasta
1 tablespoon olive oil
1-pound medium shrimp - peeled and deveined
3 tablespoons minced garlic
2 tablespoons butter
2 tablespoons grated Parmesan cheese

Nutritional Value: 411 calories per serving

DIRECTIONS

1. Cook pasta in a large pot of boiling water with olive oil until al dente.
2. Meanwhile, place the shrimp in boiling salted water for 3 to 5 minutes, just until they turn pink. Cooking time will depend on the size of the shrimp. Remove the tails, and place in a bowl of warm water.
3. In a microwave safe bowl, mix butter or olive oil and minced garlic. Microwave on high for 45 seconds, or until melted. Stir.
4. Drain pasta, and transfer to a serving dish. Toss with garlic butter and shrimp. Sprinkle with grated Parmesan cheese. Serve warm.

Pasta

Pasta and Spinach Shells

COOKING: 25 MIN

SERVES: 2

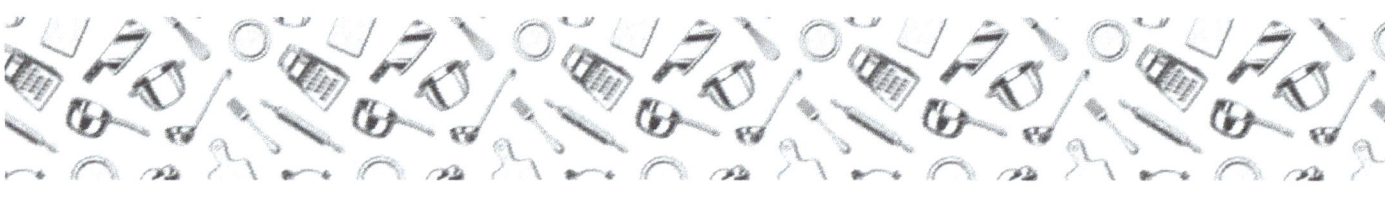

INGREDIENTS

1-pound seashell pasta
(10 ounce) package frozen chopped spinach
3 tablespoons olive oil
7 cloves garlic, minced
1 teaspoon dried red pepper flakes (optional)
Salt

Nutritional Value: 369 calories per serving

DIRECTIONS

1. Bring a large pot of lightly salted water to a boil. Add pasta and spinach and cook for 8 to 10 minutes or until pasta is al dente; drain and reserve.
2. Heat oil in a large skillet over medium heat. Add garlic and red pepper flakes; saute for 5 minutes or until the garlic turns light gold. Add cooked pasta and spinach to the skillet and mix well. Season with salt and toss; serve.

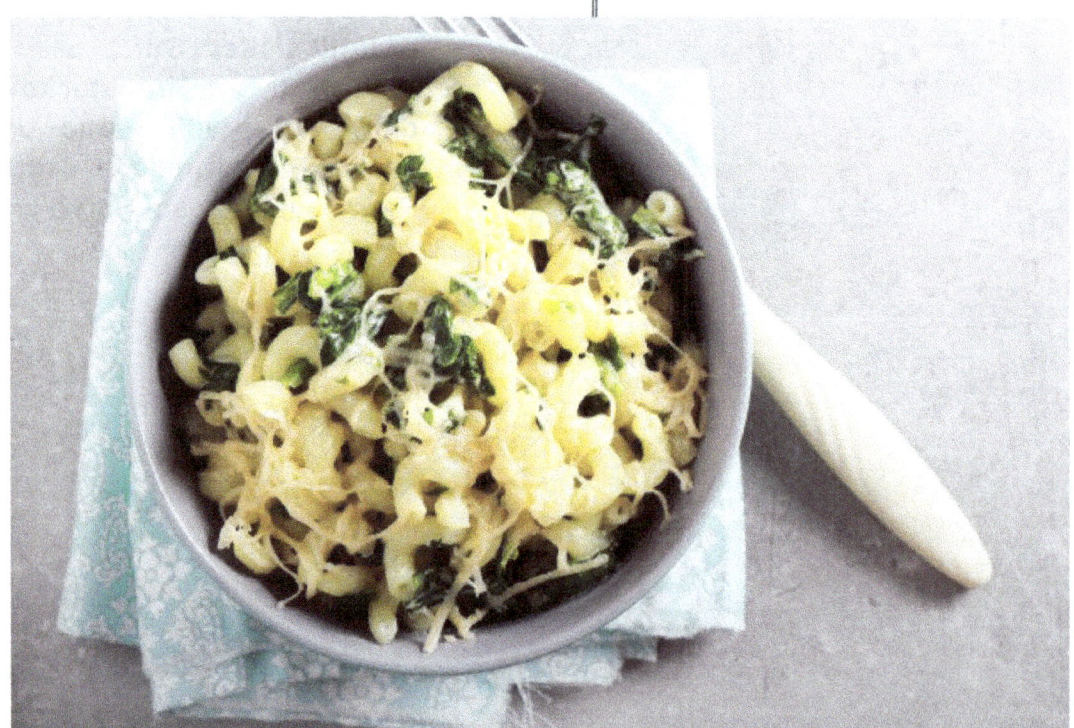

Pasta

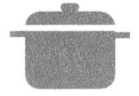

Fettucine Lasagna

COOKING: 25 MIN

SERVES: 2

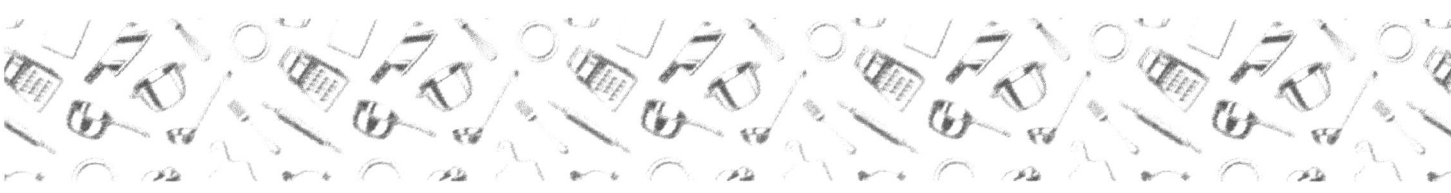

INGREDIENTS

12 ounces dry fettuccine pasta
1-pound lean ground beef (optional)
1 cup chopped onion
1 cup red bell pepper, chopped
1 tablespoon butter
1 (29 ounce) can diced tomatoes
(4 ounce) can sliced mushrooms
3 tablespoons chopped black olives
teaspoons dried oregano
1 cup shredded Cheddar cheese
1 cup shredded mozzarella cheese
1 (10.75 ounce) can condensed cream of mushroom soup
1/4 cup beef broth
1/4 cup grated Parmesan cheese

Nutritional Value: 471 calories per serving

DIRECTIONS

1. Bring a large pot of lightly salted water to a boil. Cook pasta for 8 to 10 minutes, or until al dente; drain.
2. In a large skillet, brown beef over medium heat. Drain fat from pan, and transfer meat to a bowl. In the same skillet, cook onion and bell pepper in butter until tender. Stir in tomatoes, mushrooms, olives, and beef, and season with oregano. Simmer for 10 minutes.
3. Preheat oven to 350 degrees F (175 degrees C). Lightly grease a 9x13 inch baking dish.
4. Arrange half of the cooked fettuccine in the prepared dish, top with half of the beef and vegetable mixture, and sprinkle with 1/2 cup of Cheddar cheese and 1/2 cup of mozzarella cheese. Repeat layers. Mix together soup and beef broth until smooth and pour over casserole. Sprinkle with Parmesan cheese.
5. Bake in preheated oven for 30 to 35 minutes, or until heated through

Pasta

 **Casserole from Pasta and Beans**

COOKING: 25 MIN					SERVES: 2

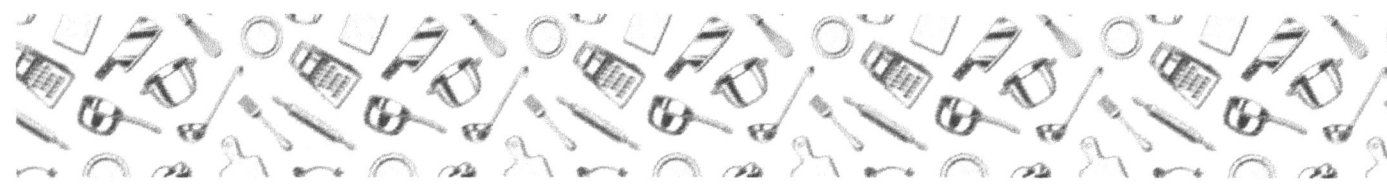

INGREDIENTS

1 (16 ounce) package seashell pasta
tablespoons olive oil
1 medium onion, peeled and diced
3 cloves garlic, minced
1/2 green bell pepper, chopped
1/2 red bell pepper, chopped
1 jalapeno pepper, minced (optional)
1 (14.5 ounce) can diced tomatoes with juice
1 (15 ounce) can garbanzo beans
1 teaspoon basil
1 teaspoon dried oregano 1 teaspoon ground paprika
1 teaspoon ground cumin
1 teaspoon ground coriander salt to taste
Pepper
1/2 cup shredded mozzarella cheese

Nutritional Value: 214 calories per serving

DIRECTIONS

1. Preheat oven to 350 degrees F (175 degrees C). Oil a 9x13 inch baking dish.
2. Bring a large pot of lightly salted water to a boil. Cook pasta in boiling water for 8 to 10 minutes, or until al dente. Drain.
3. Heat olive oil in a skillet over medium heat. Cook onion in oil until soft, then add garlic and red and green peppers. Stir in jalapeno, if desired. Continue cooking for 2 more minutes. Stir in tomatoes and garbanzo beans. Season with basil, oregano, paprika, cumin, coriander, and salt and pepper. Simmer with 5 minutes. Remove from heat and stir in pasta. Transfer to prepared baking dish, and top with cheese.
4. Bake in preheated oven for 30 to 40 minutes, or until cheese is melted and bubbly.

Pasta

Spinach and Feta Pasta

COOKING: 25 MIN SERVES: 2

INGREDIENTS

1 (8 ounce) package penne pasta
2 tablespoons olive oil
1/2 cup chopped onion
1 clove garlic, minced
3 cups chopped tomatoes
1 cup sliced fresh mushrooms
2 cups spinach leaves, packed salt and pepper to taste
1 pinch red pepper flakes
8 ounces feta cheese, crumbled

Nutritional Value: 147 calories per serving

DIRECTIONS

1. Bring a large pot of lightly salted water to a boil. Cook pasta in boiling water until al dente; drain.
2. Meanwhile, heat olive oil in a large skillet over medium-high heat; add onion and garlic and cook until golden brown. Mix in tomatoes, mushrooms, and spinach. Season with salt, pepper, and red pepper flakes. Cook 2 minutes more, until tomatoes are heated through and spinach is wilted. Reduce heat to medium, stir in pasta and feta cheese, and cook until heated through

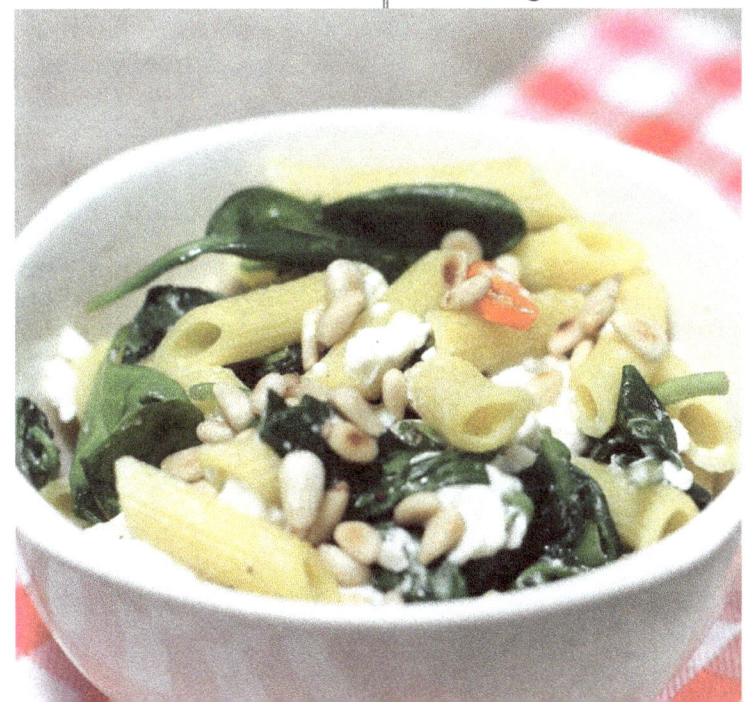

Pasta

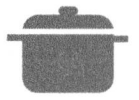 Lasagna with Mushrooms

COOKING: 25 MIN   SERVES: 2

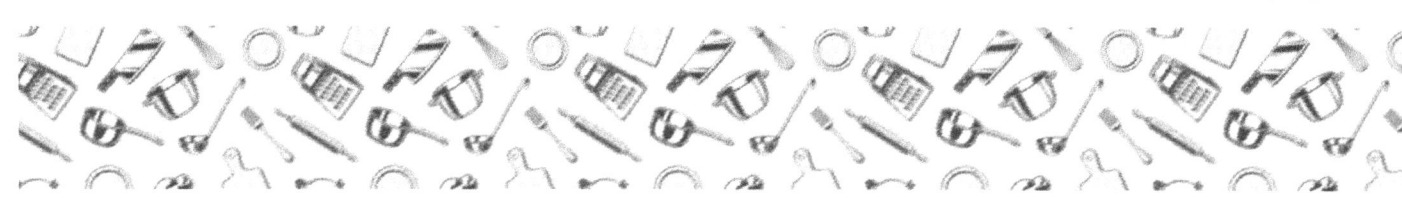

INGREDIENTS

1/4-pound lean ground beef
1/2 cup fat-free small curd cottage cheese
1 egg
1 tablespoon finely chopped green onion
1 tablespoon chopped fresh parsley
Salt
Pepper
1/4 cup prepared pasta sauce, divided
6 large fresh mushrooms, or more as needed, stems removed
1/4 cup shredded mozzarella cheese, divided

Nutritional Value: 469 calories per serving

DIRECTIONS

1. Preheat oven to 375 degrees F (190 degrees C). Spray an 8x8-inch baking dish with cooking spray.
2. Cook and stir the ground beef in a skillet over medium heat, breaking it apart as it cooks, until the meat is no longer pink, about 10 minutes. Mix together the cottage cheese, egg, green onion, parsley, and salt and pepper in a bowl until the mixture is well Mixd. Stir in the cooked ground beef.
3. Place the mushrooms, hollow sides up, close together in the prepared baking dish. Spoon about 1 tablespoon of the cheese filling into the cavity of each mushroom and allow remaining filling to overflow between mushrooms.
4. Bake in the preheated oven until the cheese filling is set, about 15 minutes. Remove dish from oven and spread the pasta sauce evenly over the mushrooms. Sprinkle an even layer of mozzarella cheese over the sauce, return the dish to the oven, and broil until the cheese is bubbling and beginning to brown, about 5 more minutes. Let the mushrooms stand 5 minutes before serving..

Pasta

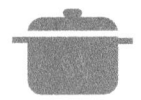

Carbonara Spaghetti vol.1

COOKING: 25 MIN   SERVES: 2

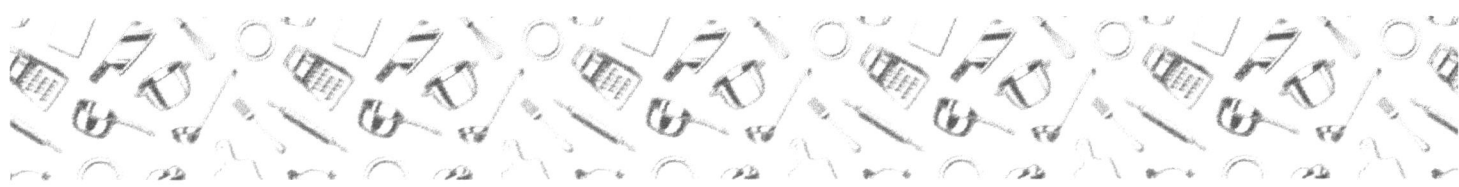

INGREDIENTS

1-pound spaghetti
1 tablespoon olive oil 8 slices bacon, diced
1 tablespoon olive oil 1 onion, chopped
clove garlic, minced
1/4 cup dry white wine (optional)
4 eggs
1/2 cup grated Parmesan cheese
1 pinch salt and black pepper to taste
tablespoons chopped fresh parsley
2 tablespoons grated Parmesan cheese

Nutritional Value: 471 calories per serving

DIRECTIONS

1. In a large pot of boiling salted water, cook spaghetti pasta until al dente. Drain well. Toss with 1 tablespoon of olive oil and set aside.
2. Meanwhile in a large skillet, cook chopped bacon until slightly crisp; remove and drain onto paper towels. Reserve 2 tablespoons of bacon fat; add remaining 1 tablespoon olive oil, and heat in reused large skillet. Add chopped onion and cook over medium heat until onion is translucent. Add minced garlic and cook 1 minute more.
3. Add wine if desired; cook one more minute.
4. Return cooked bacon to pan; add cooked and drained spaghetti. Toss to coat and heat through, adding more olive oil if it seems dry or is sticking together. Add beaten eggs and cook, tossing constantly with tongs or large fork until eggs are barely set. Quickly add 1/2 cup Parmesan cheese and toss again. Add salt and pepper to taste (remember that bacon and Parmesan are very salty).
5. Serve immediately with chopped parsley sprinkled on top, and extra Parmesan cheese at table.

Pasta

Turkey Pasta

COOKING: 25 MIN

SERVES: 2

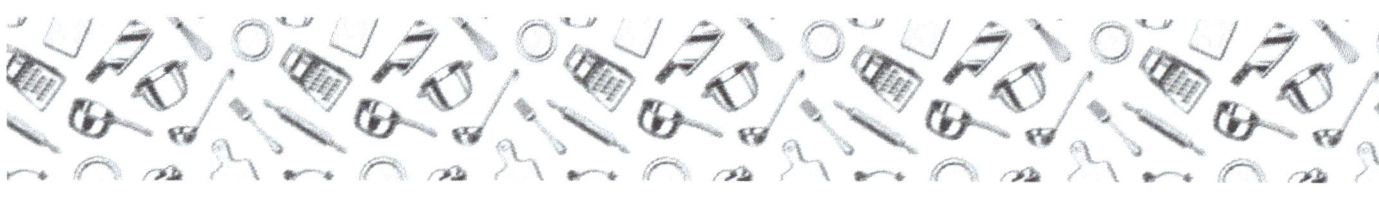

INGREDIENTS

1/2 (16 ounce) package whole-wheat spaghetti
Olive oil
1 small red onion, thinly sliced
1 green bell pepper, chopped
1-pound cubed cooked turkey
1 (26 ounce) jar spaghetti sauce
1 cup shredded mozzarella cheese

Nutritional Value: 236 calories per serving

DIRECTIONS

1. Fill a large pot with lightly salted water and bring to a rolling boil over high heat. Once the water is boiling, stir in the spaghetti, and return to a boil. Cook the pasta uncovered, stirring occasionally, until the pasta has cooked through, but is still firm to the bite, about 12 minutes. Drain well in a colander set in the sink.
2. Meanwhile, heat the olive oil in a large saucepan or Dutch oven over medium heat. Stir in the onion and green pepper. Cook and stir until the onion has softened and turned translucent, about 5 minutes. Stir in the turkey and spaghetti sauce. Bring to a simmer over medium-high heat, then cover, and reduce heat to medium-low. Cook until the sauce is hot.
3. Once the spaghetti has been cooked and drained, stir it into the hot sauce along with the mozzarella cheese. Stir until the cheese melts, then serve.

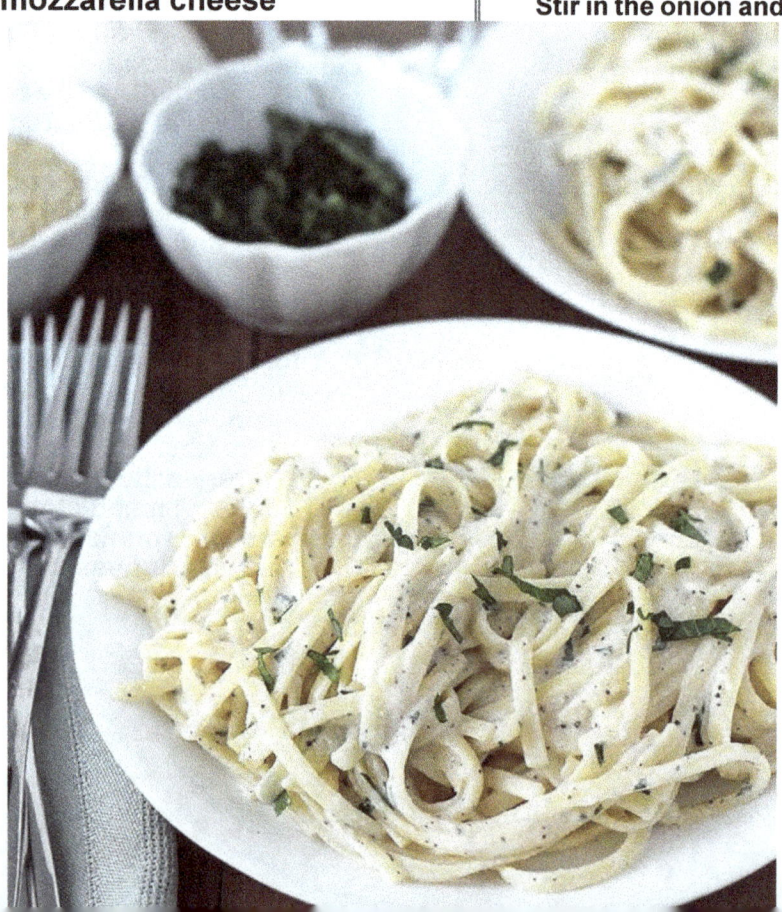

Pasta

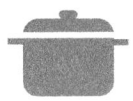

Fettuccine with Yogurt and Shrimp

COOKING: 25 MIN   SERVES: 2

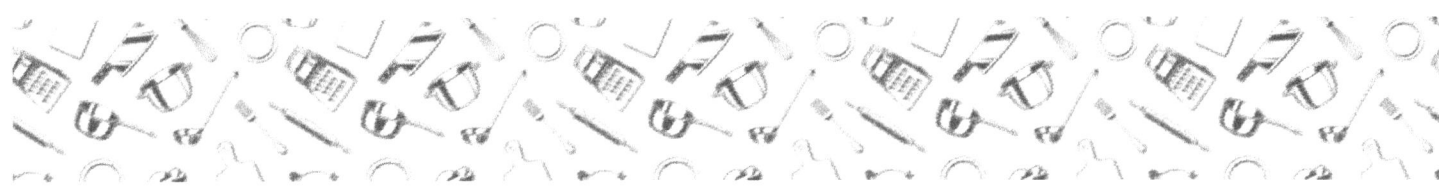

INGREDIENTS

16 ounces dry fettuccine pasta
2 tablespoons butter
1 1/2 pounds medium shrimp - peeled and deveined
salt and pepper to taste
2 teaspoons paprika
1 red bell pepper, chopped
1 green bell pepper, sliced
1 tablespoon minced shallots
1 teaspoon chopped garlic
2 tablespoons brandy
1/2 cup sour cream
1 cup plain yogurt
4 tablespoons chopped fresh cilantro

Nutritional Value: 452 calories per serving

DIRECTIONS

1. Bring a large pot of lightly salted water to a boil. Add pasta and cook for 8 to 10 minutes or until al dente. Drain and set aside.
2. Heat butter or olive oil in a large skillet. Add the shrimp, salt and pepper to taste and paprika. Stir with a wooden spatula. When the shrimp become pink (it should take 2 to 3 minutes), remove them with a slotted spoon, leaving the cooking liquid in the skillet.
3. Add red and green bell peppers, shallots, garlic and salt and pepper to taste. Cook, stirring, about 3 to 4 minutes over medium high heat. Add cognac and shrimp. Cook over medium heat for 2 more minutes.
4. Add sour cream and yogurt and blend all together. Add cilantro and bring to a simmer for about 30 seconds. Do not boil or sauce will separate. Serve over cooked fettuccine

Pasta

Fagioli Pasta

COOKING: 25 MIN   SERVES: 2

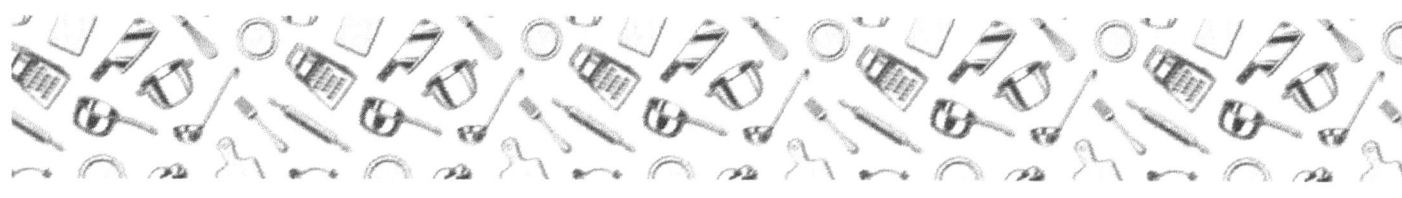

INGREDIENTS

2 cups cranberry beans
6 cups cold water
1/2 cup white wine
2 cups beef broth
4 1/2 cups chicken broth
3 cloves crushed garlic
tablespoon tomato paste
tablespoons chopped fresh parsley
(8 ounce) package farfalle pasta
1/3 cup grated Parmesan cheese
1 tablespoon olive oil
tablespoons grated Parmesan cheese

Nutritional Value: 326 calories per serving

DIRECTIONS

1. In a large pot, place cranberry beans and water. Bring to a boil. Cover pot and turn heat off. Allow to stand for one hour on burner.
2. Drain beans and return to large cooking pot. Add wine, beef broth, and chicken broth. Bring to boil, cover and simmer for 30 minutes.
3. Puree half of the beans. Return to the pot. Add the garlic, tomato paste, parsley, and farfalle pasta. Simmer gently, uncovered, for 25 to 30 minutes, or until pasta is tender and soup is thick. Stir in the grated Parmesan cheese. Garnish with drizzled olive oil, and additional grated Parmesan cheese...

Pasta

Macaroni with 4 types of Cheese

COOKING: 25 MIN   SERVES: 2

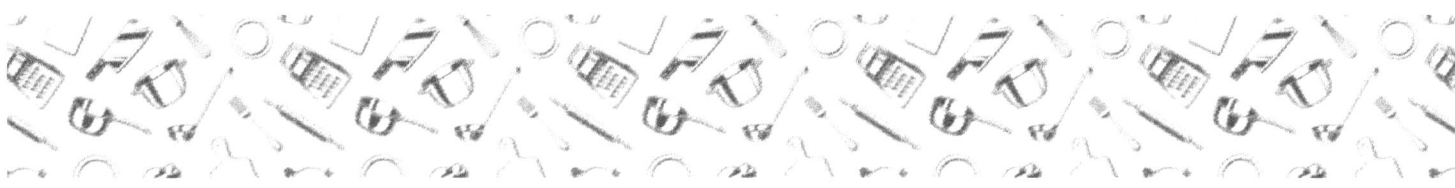

INGREDIENTS

1 tablespoon olive oil
1 (16 ounce) package elbow macaroni
9 tablespoons butter
1/2 cup shredded Muenster cheese
1/2 cup shredded Cheddar cheese
1/2 cup shredded sharp Cheddar cheese
1/2 cup shredded Monterey Jack cheese
1 1/2 cups half-and-half
8 ounces cubed processed cheese food
2 eggs, beaten
1/4 teaspoon salt
1/8 teaspoon ground black pepper

Nutritional Value: 258 calories per serving

DIRECTIONS

1. Bring a large pot of lightly salted water to a boil. Add the oil and the pasta and cook for 8 to 10 minutes or until al dente; drain well and return to cooking pot.
2. In a small saucepan over medium heat, melt 8 tablespoons butter; stir into the macaroni.
3. In a large bowl, Mix the Muenster cheese, mild and sharp Cheddar cheeses, and Monterey Jack cheese; mix well.
4. Preheat oven to 350 degrees F (175 degrees C)
5. Add the half and half, 1 1/2 cups of cheese mixture, cubed processed cheese food, and eggs to macaroni; mix together and season with salt and pepper. Transfer to a lightly greased deep 2 1/2-quart casserole dish. Sprinkle with the remaining 1/2 cup of cheese mixture and 1 tablespoon of butter.
6. Bake in preheated oven for 35 minutes or until hot and bubbling around the edges; serve...

Pasta

Meatball and Pasta Dish

COOKING: 25 MIN　　　　　　　　　　　　　　　　　　　　SERVES: 2

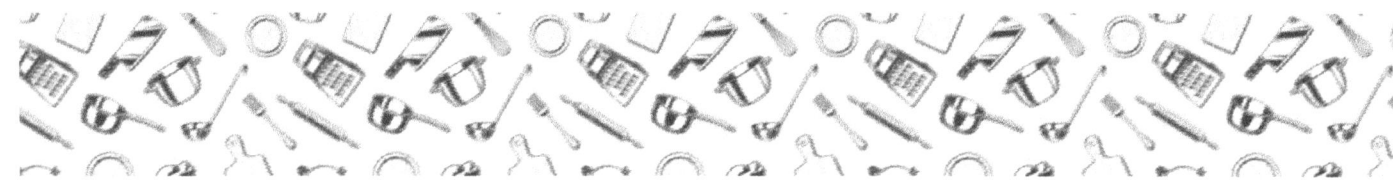

INGREDIENTS

For the meatballs:
1/2-pound lean ground beef
1/2-pound bulk Italian sausage
1/3 cup grated Parmesan cheese
1/3 cup seasoned breadcrumbs
1/4 cup milk
1 egg
3 tablespoons dried parsley
1 clove garlic, minced
1/8 teaspoon ground black pepper
2 tablespoons minced onion
1 tablespoon olive oil, or as needed
For the soup:
1 tablespoon butter
large carrot, chopped
2 stalks celery, chopped
3/4 cup chopped yellow onion
7 cups beef stock
3 tablespoons Italian-style tomato paste
1 (14.5 ounce) can chopped tomatoes
1/2 teaspoon salt, or to taste
1/4 teaspoon ground black pepper, or to taste
6 ounces uncooked tri-color wagon wheel pasta

DIRECTIONS

1. Mix together in a bowl the ground beef, sausage, Parmesan cheese, breadcrumbs, milk, egg, parsley, garlic, pepper, and onion. Roll into small meatballs, about 1 to 2 teaspoons each. Heat olive oil in a large skillet over medium-high heat. Brown meatballs in batches and drain on paper towels, wiping out pan between batches and adding more oil as needed.
2. Melt butter in a large pot over medium heat. Add carrots, celery, and onion and cook until slightly softened, about 8 minutes. Stir in the meatballs, stock, tomato paste, tomatoes, salt and pepper.
3. Bring to a boil, then reduce heat to low. Simmer for 30 minutes. Skim fat from surface.
4. Bring a large pot of salted water to a boil. Add pasta and cook until al dente, 8 to 10 minutes. Drain. Cover and set aside.

Nutritional Value: 356 calories per serving

Pasta

Spinach Noodles

COOKING: 25 MIN

SERVES: 2

INGREDIENTS

1 (16 ounce) package spinach spaghetti pasta
1/2 cup butter, divided
5 pollock fillets
1 small onion, diced
1 (7 ounce) can escargot, drained
2 cloves garlic, chopped
1 tablespoon chopped fresh parsley
1 teaspoon dried oregano
1/2 teaspoon dried basil
1/4 cup grated Parmesan cheese for topping

Nutritional Value: 541 calories per serving

DIRECTIONS

1. Bring a large pot of lightly salted water to a boil. Add the spaghetti, and cook until tender, about 7 minutes. Drain, stir in a tablespoon of butter, and set aside.
2. Melt 1 tablespoon of butter in a skillet over medium heat. Add the onion and garlic and cook until lightly browned. Lay the pollock fillets in the skillet, and cook until golden on each side, about 5 minutes. When the fillets are starting to be done, break them into pieces with a fork or spatula.
3. Add the remaining butter to the skillet and stir in the escargot. Cook and stir for about minutes. Escargot cooks fast like shrimp, so watch it. Remove from the heat, and season with parsley, oregano and basil. Top with a sprinkling of Parmesan cheese

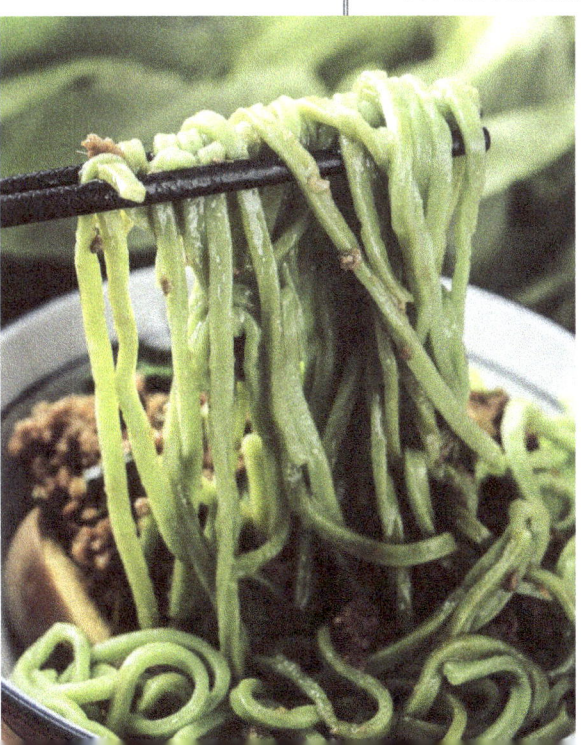

Pasta

Chicken Cacciatore and Pasta

COOKING: 25 MIN

SERVES: 2

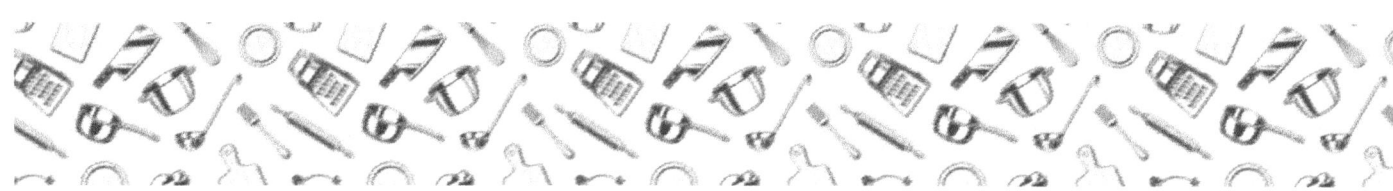

INGREDIENTS

1 tablespoon olive oil
4 skinless, boneless chicken breast halves
1 3/4 cups chicken stock
1 teaspoon dried oregano leaves, crushed
1 teaspoon garlic powder
1 (14.5 ounce) can diced tomatoes
1 small green pepper, slice into 2-inch long strips
1 medium onion, slice into wedges
1/4 teaspoon ground black pepper
1/2 cups uncooked medium shell-shaped pasta

Nutritional Value: 321 calories per serving

DIRECTIONS

1. Heat the oil in a 10-inch skillet over medium-high heat. Add the chicken and cook for 10 minutes or until it's well browned on both sides.
2. Stir the stock, oregano, garlic powder, tomatoes, green pepper, onion and black pepper in the skillet and heat to a boil. Stir in the pasta. Reduce the heat to low. Cover and cook for 15 minutes or until the pasta is tender...

Pasta

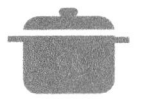

Bow tie Pasta and Beef

COOKING: 25 MIN

SERVES: 2

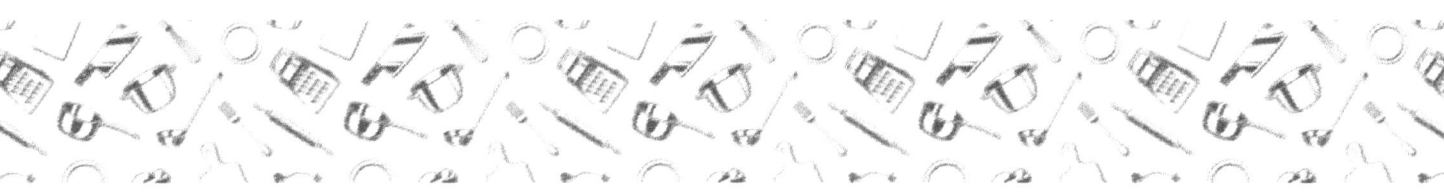

INGREDIENTS

1 1/2 cups bow-tie pasta (farfalle)
1-pound ground beef
3 cloves garlic, minced
2 cups chopped fresh tomatoes
3/4 teaspoon salt
1/4 teaspoon black pepper
2 tablespoons chopped fresh basil
3 tablespoons grated Parmesan cheese

Nutritional Value: 325 calories per serving

DIRECTIONS

1. Fill a large pot with lightly salted water and bring to a rolling boil over high heat. Once the water is boiling, stir in the bow-tie pasta and return to a boil. Cook the pasta uncovered, stirring occasionally, until the pasta has cooked through, but is still firm to the bite, about 12 minutes. Drain well in a colander set in the sink.
2. In a large skillet over medium heat, cook the ground beef until browned and crumbly, about 10 minutes; drain off excess fat. Stir in garlic and cook for 5 minutes, stirring frequently. Stir in tomatoes, salt, and pepper. Cook, stirring occasionally, until tomatoes are soft, about 5 minutes.
3. Place the bow-tie pasta into a large serving dish and pour the ground beef mixture over the pasta. Sprinkle on the chopped basil. Toss lightly to Mix, and sprinkle with Parmesan cheese before serving.

Pasta

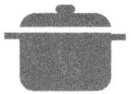

4 of July Pasta

COOKING: 25 MIN   SERVES: 2

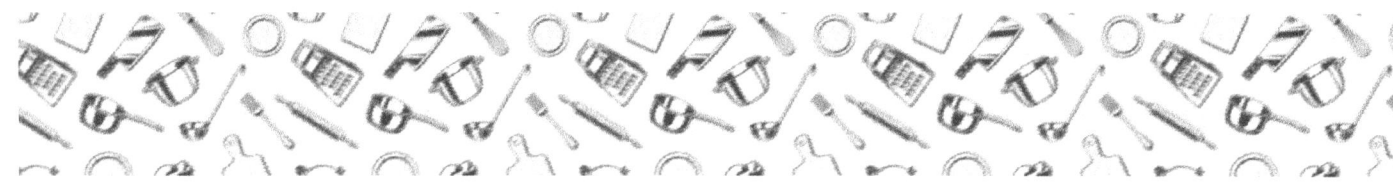

INGREDIENTS

Dressing
1/4 cup mayonnaise
1/4 cup sour cream
1/4 cup crumbled blue cheese
1 1/2 teaspoons milk
1/2 teaspoon salt
1/2 teaspoon white vinegar
1/4 teaspoon garlic powder
1/4 teaspoon pepper
1/2 teaspoon honey mustard
1/8 teaspoon cayenne pepper
Salad:
2 1/2 cups uncooked penne or medium tube pasta
1 garlic clove, minced
3/4 teaspoon minced fresh basil
2 tablespoons olive oil
1 1/2 cups fresh cauliflowerets
1 cup cherry tomatoes, halved
3 green onions, chopped
1/4 cup chopped sweet red pepper
4 ounces mozzarella cheese, slice into 1-inch strips
2 tablespoons grated Parmesan cheese

Nutritional Value: 478 calories per serving

DIRECTIONS

1. In a small bowl, Mix the dressing Ingredients; set aside. Meanwhile cook pasta according to package Instructions; rinse in cold water and drain. Transfer to a large bowl.
2. Meanwhile, in a large skillet, sauté garlic and basil in oil until garlic is tender. Pour over pasta. Add the cauliflower, tomatoes, green onions, red pepper, cheese and dressing; toss to coat. Cover and refrigerate until serving.

Pasta

Chicken and Pasta with Balsamic Vinegar

COOKING: 25 MIN   SERVES: 2

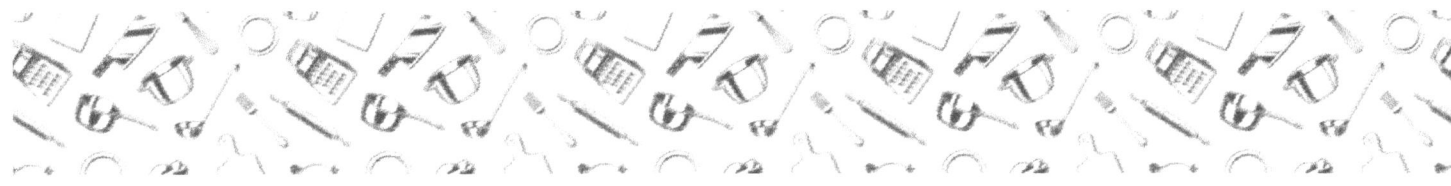

INGREDIENTS

3 cloves garlic, minced
2 ounces fresh basil leaves
1/2 cup olive oil
1/2 cup balsamic vinegar
6 skinless, boneless chicken breast halves
1 tablespoon salt
1 1/2 teaspoons ground black pepper
1-pound penne pasta
2 pints grape tomatoes, halved
1/4 cup olive oil
1/4 cup balsamic vinegar
Salt and pepper to taste

Nutritional Value: 369 calories per serving

DIRECTIONS

1. Mince garlic cloves in food processor or blender. Add 1/3 of the basil leaves to the processor, and chop until fine. Pour in 1/2 cup of olive oil and continue to process until mixture turns light yellow with flecks of basil. Add the balsamic vinegar; process just until Mixd.
2. Place the chicken breasts in a large zip-top storage bag along with 1 tablespoon salt, 1 1/2 teaspoons pepper, and the contents of the food processor. Squeeze air out of bag and seal. Allow chicken to marinate for 2 hours, or up to overnight, turning occasionally.
3. Preheat the oven to 300 degrees F (150 degrees C).
4. Brown chicken in a large skillet over large heat, about 4 to 5 minutes per side. Transfer chicken to a large baking dish, and place in the oven until cooked through, about 15 to 20 minutes. Remove chicken from oven, slice into 1/4-inch strips, and return to baking dish to absorb cooking juices. Keep warm.
5. While chicken is baking, bring a large pot of water to a boil over high heat. Boil the pasta until cooked through, but still firm to the bite, about 11 minutes. Drain well. Stir the chicken and the juices from the baking dish into the hot pasta.
6. Thinly slice the remaining basil leaves, and place in a large serving bowl along with the tomatoes. Stir in 1/4 cup olive oil, 1/4 cup balsamic vinegar, and salt and pepper to taste. Top basil and tomatoes with the hot pasta, sauce, and chicken; toss to mix

Pasta

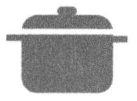

Fettuccini Alfredo with Chicken

COOKING: 25 MIN   SERVES: 2

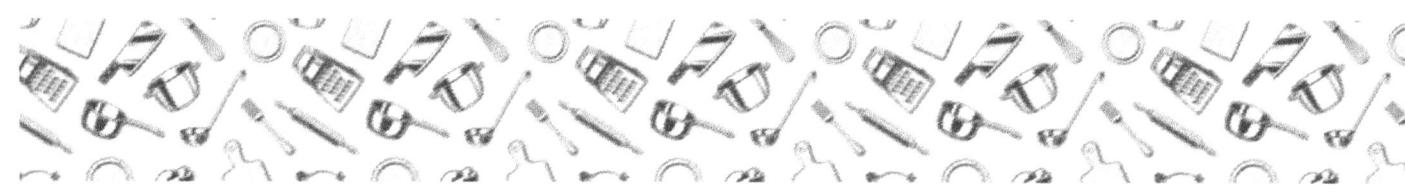

INGREDIENTS

6 skinless, boneless chicken breast halves - slice into cubes
6 tablespoons butter, divided
4 cloves garlic, minced, divided
1 tablespoon Italian seasoning
1-pound fettuccini pasta
1 onion, diced
1 (8 ounce) package sliced mushrooms
1/3 cup all-purpose flour
1 tablespoon salt
3/4 teaspoon ground white pepper
3 cups milk
1 cup half-and-half
3/4 cup grated Parmesan cheese
8 ounces shredded Colby- Monterey Jack cheese
3 roma (plum) tomatoes, diced
1/2 cup sour cream

Nutritional Value: 256 calories per serving

DIRECTIONS

1. In a large skillet over medium heat Mix chicken, 2 tablespoons butter, garlic and Italian seasoning. Cook until chicken is no longer pink inside. Remove from skillet and set aside.
2. Bring a large pot of lightly salted water to a boil. Add pasta and cook for 8 to 10 minutes or until al dente; drain.
3. Meanwhile, melt 4 tablespoons butter in the skillet. Sauté onion, 2 tablespoons garlic and mushrooms until onions are transparent.
4. Stir in flour, salt and pepper; cook 2 minutes. Slowly add milk and half-and-half, stirring until smooth and creamy. Stir in Parmesan and Colby-Monterey Jack cheeses; stir until cheese is melted. Stir in chicken mixture, tomatoes and sour cream. Serve over cooked fettuccini.

Pasta

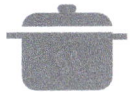

Manicotti

COOKING: 25 MIN

SERVES: 2

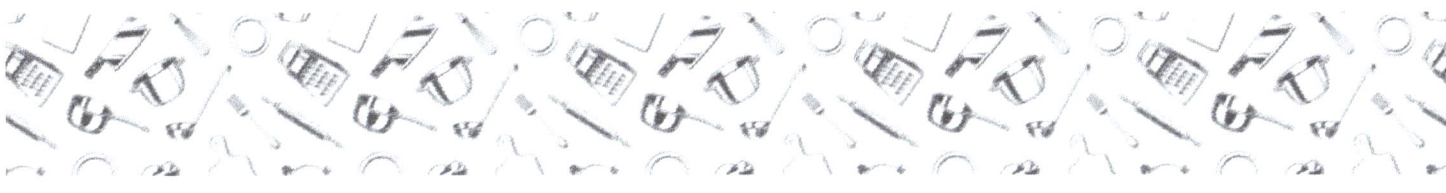

INGREDIENTS

1 lb. Italian sweet sausage links
1 lb. ground beef
1 medium onion, chopped
2 16 oz. cans tomato puree
1 6 oz. can tomato paste
1 tsp. sugar
1/2 tsp. pepper
2 tbsp. parsley, chopped
basil
salt
1 8 oz. package manicotti shells
4 cups ricotta cheese
1 8 oz. package mozzarella cheese
Parmesan cheese

Nutritional Value: 254 calories per serving

DIRECTIONS

1. In covered 5-quart Dutch oven. Over medium heat, in 1/4 cup water, cook sausage links 5 minutes. Uncover, brown well, drain on paper towel.
2. Spoon fat from Dutch oven. over medium heat brown ground beef and onions, stir in tomato puree, paste, sugar, pepper, 1 tsp. basil, 1 tsp. salt, 1 cup water; simmer, covered 45 minutes.
3. Cut sausage into bite-size pieces; add to mixture and cook 15 minutes, stirring occasionally. Meanwhile, cook manicotti as label directs; drain. Preheat oven to 375 degrees.
4. In a large bowl, combine ricotta and mozzarella (diced) cheeses, parsley, 3/4 tsp. basil, 1/2 tsp salt: stuff into shells.
5. Spoon half of meat sauce into 13" x 9" baking dish. Place half of shells over sauce in one layer. Spoon remaining sauce, except 3/4 cup, over shells, top with remaining shells in one layer.
6. Spoon reserved meat sauce over top. Sprinkle with parmesan. Bake 30 minutes

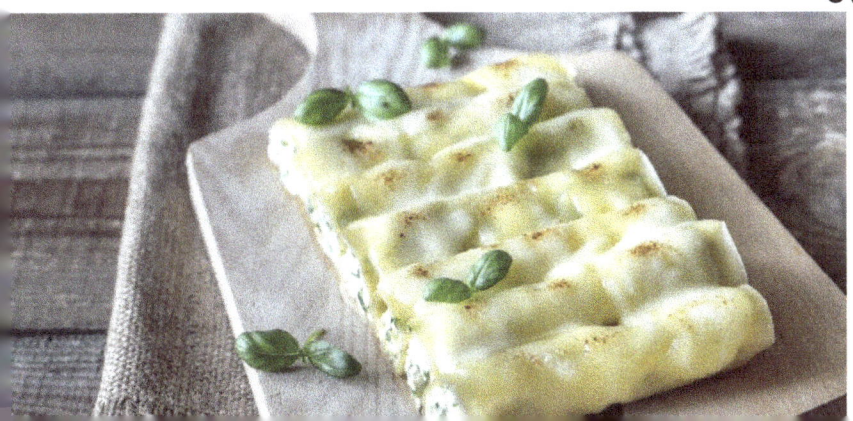

Pasta

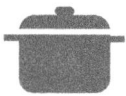 **Cheddar Macaroni with Bacon and Thyme**

COOKING: 25 MIN   SERVES: 2

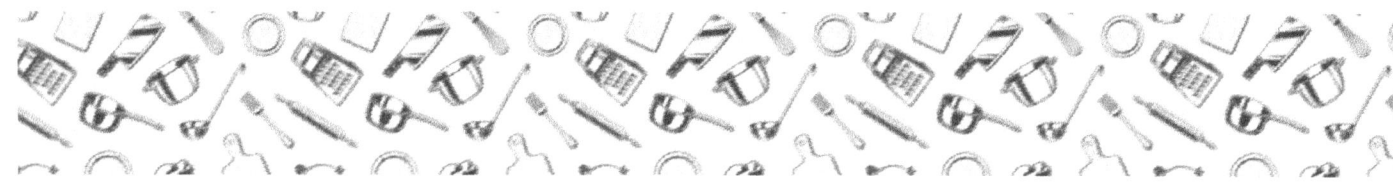

INGREDIENTS

1 tablespoon grated Parmesan cheese, or as needed
1-pound mezze (short) penne pasta
1-pound thick sliced bacon, slice into
1/2-inch pieces
1/4 cup butter
1 small onion, chopped
1/3 cup all-purpose flour
4 cups milk
1 teaspoon dried thyme leaves sea salt and cracked black pepper to taste
1/4 cup grated Parmesan cheese
3 1/2 cups shredded sharp white Cheddar cheese, divided

Nutritional Value: 478 calories per serving

DIRECTIONS

1. Preheat oven to 350 degrees F (175 degrees C). Grease a 9x13-inch baking dish, and sprinkle 1 tablespoon Parmesan cheese around the inside of the dish.
2. Fill a large pot with lightly salted water and bring to a rolling boil. Once the water is boiling, stir in the penne, and return to a boil. Cook the penne uncovered, stirring occasionally, until the pasta has cooked through, but is still firm to the bite, about 11 minutes. Drain well in a colander set in the sink.
3. Place the bacon pieces into a large, deep skillet, and cook over medium-high heat, stirring occasionally, until evenly browned, about 10 minutes. Drain the bacon slices on a paper towel-lined plate.
4. Retain 1/4 cup of bacon drippings. Set the bacon pieces aside.
5. Melt butter and bacon drippings together in a large saucepan over medium heat, and cook and stir the onion until translucent, about 5 minutes. Whisk in the flour, stirring frequently until the mixture forms a smooth paste. Whisk in the milk, a little at a time, and bring the mixture to a simmer, whisking constantly until thickened. Stir in the thyme, salt, and pepper, and then whisk in 1/4 cup Parmesan and 3 cups Cheddar cheese, stirring constantly until the Cheddar cheese has melted and the sauce is smooth and thick
6. Stir the cooked penne pasta into the cheese sauce, then lightly mix in the cooked bacon. Spread the mixture into the prepared baking dish and sprinkle 1/2 cup Cheddar cheese over the top. Cover the dish with foil.
7. Bake in the preheated oven until the pasta is hot and bubbling, about 25 minutes. Remove the dish from the oven and turn on the broiler. Remove the foil and broil the dish until the cheese topping is browned and crisp, about 5 minutes.

Pasta

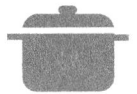

Bang Noodles

COOKING: 25 MIN

SERVES: 2

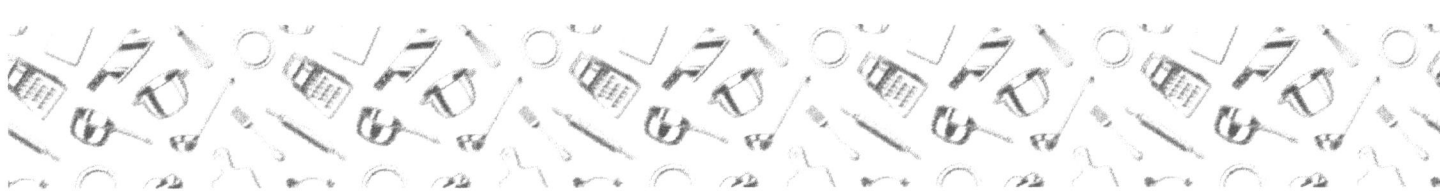

INGREDIENTS

1/2-pound Chinese wheat noodles or whole-wheat spaghetti
1/3 cup sesame ginger dressing
1/4 cup Thai-style sweet chili sauce
3 tablespoons creamy peanut butter
1 medium orange, zested and juiced
1 teaspoon hot chili oil, or to taste (sriracha may be substituted)
2 cups shredded chicken
2 cups broccoli coleslaw mix
1 hothouse (seedless) cucumber, slice in 1/2-inch dice
1 small red bell pepper, slice in 1/4-inch dice
1/2 cup chopped fresh cilantro
Salt
Pepper
Garnish:
Crisp, curly lettuce leaves
tablespoons chopped fresh cilantro
1/4 cup chopped peanuts

Nutritional Value: 300 calories per serving

DIRECTIONS

1. Bring 4-quarts of salted water to a boil over high heat; add pasta and cook until al dente stage is reached. Drain pasta; rinse with cold water and return to pan.
2. Place salad dressing, chili sauce, peanut butter, orange juice and zest in a small bowl; whisk to Mix. Stir in 1 teaspoon chili oil. Taste. If more heat is desired, add additional chili oil, a teaspoon at a time, until seasoned to taste - exercise caution as chili oil is very hot.
3. Pour sauce over noodles. Add chicken, broccoli slaw, cucumbers, bell pepper, and 1/2 cup cilantro; toss to Mix. Add salt and pepper to taste. Line a platter with lettuce leaves, top with noodles and garnish with reserved 2 tablespoons cilantro and chopped peanuts. Serve at room temperature.

Pasta

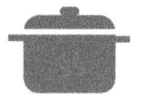 Tarragon Chicken Pasta

COOKING: 25 MIN   SERVES: 2

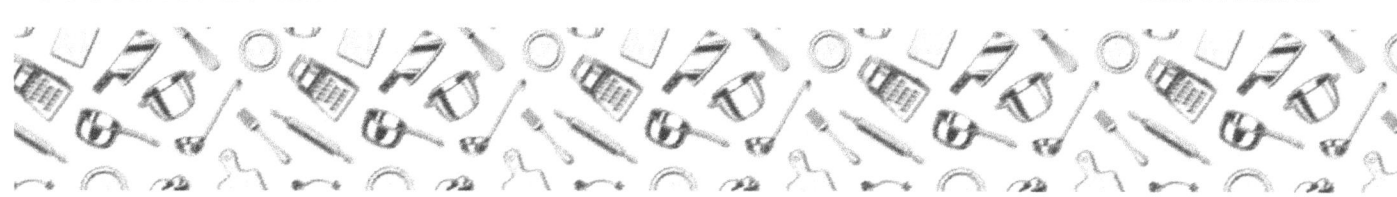

INGREDIENTS

1-pound dry whole-wheat noodles
5 tablespoons butter
3 shallots, thinly sliced
1 red bell pepper, julienned
1 yellow bell pepper, julienned
1 clove garlic, minced
1-pound skinless, boneless chicken breast halves - slice into strips
1 1/2 teaspoons dried tarragon
1/4 teaspoon salt
1/4 teaspoon ground black pepper
3/4 cup half-and-half cream
1 1/2 cups shredded Monterey Jack cheese
1/4 cup grated Parmesan cheese

Nutritional Value: 236 calories per serving

DIRECTIONS

1. Bring a large pot of lightly salted water to a boil. Place noodles in the pot, cook 8 to 10 minutes, until al dente, and drain.
2. Melt the butter in a large skillet over medium heat. Stir in the shallots, red bell pepper, yellow bell pepper, and garlic. Cook 5 minutes, until tender but crisp. Remove vegetables from skillet and set aside.
3. Place the chicken in the skillet. Season with tarragon, salt, and pepper. Cook 10 minutes, or until juices run clear.
4. Return the vegetables to the skillet with the chicken. Mix in the half and half, Monterey Jack cheese, and Parmesan cheese. Continue cooking 5 minutes, until cheese is melted. Serve over the cooked noodles.

Pasta

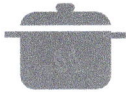 Pasta with Vegetables, Tahini and Yogurt Sauce

COOKING: 25 MIN   SERVES: 2

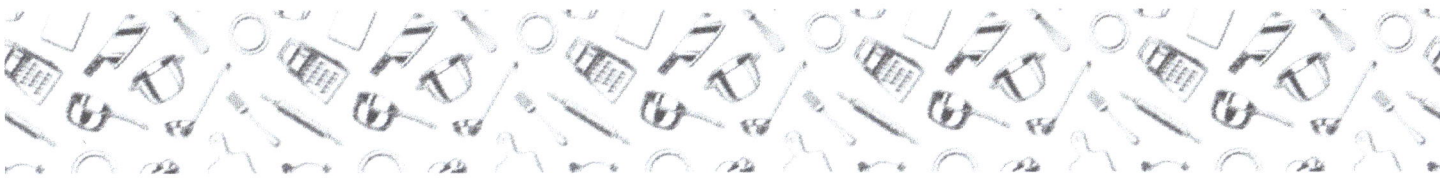

INGREDIENTS

1 (16 ounce) package wide egg noodles
3 tablespoons tahini
1 lemon, juiced
1 1/4 cups water
3 cloves garlic, minced
1 cup yogurt, drained
1/4 teaspoon hot pepper sauce
1/4 cup olive oil
1 large red bell pepper, thinly sliced
1 zucchini, thinly sliced salt to taste
ground black pepper to taste

Nutritional Value: 258 calories per serving

DIRECTIONS

Cook noodles in a large pot of boiling water until al dente. Drain.
2. Meanwhile, mix together tahini, lemon juice, and water until smooth. Add garlic, yogurt, and pepper sauce.
3. In a medium skillet, heat oil over medium high heat. Saute red pepper and zucchini in oil for 2 to 3 minutes, or until tender crisp. Add tahini sauce, and heat through. Season to taste with salt and pepper. Do not boil or overcook: this sauce curdles easily. Toss noodles with sauce.

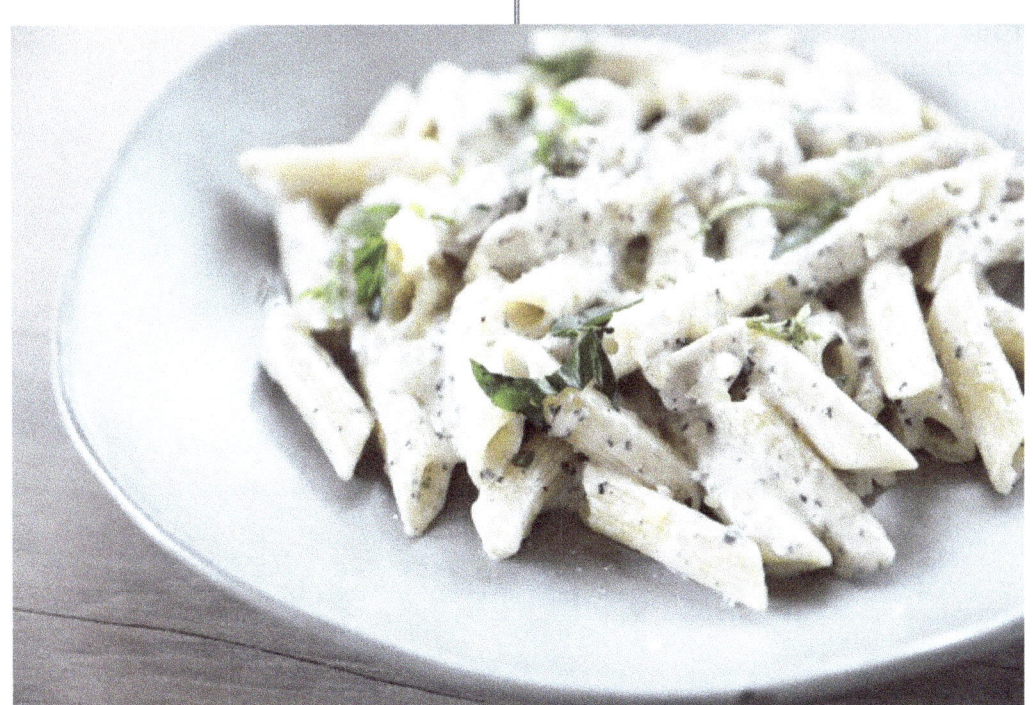

Pasta

Three Cheese Pasta

COOKING: 25 MIN   SERVES: 2

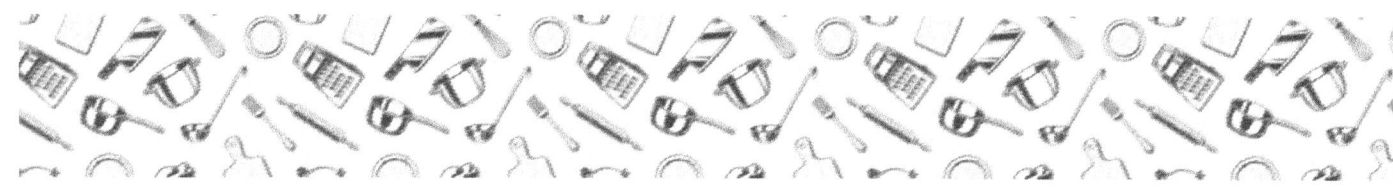

INGREDIENTS

1 (16 ounce) jar salsa
1 (8 ounce) can no-salt-added tomato sauce
1/2 cup shredded carrots
1/2 cup shredded zucchini
1/2 cup sliced fresh mushrooms
1/4 cup chopped green onions
1 garlic clove, minced
1 teaspoon canola oil
1 (15 ounce) container reduced-fat ricotta cheese
1/4 cup grated Parmesan cheese
1/4 cup shredded part-skim mozzarella cheese
1/4 cup egg substitute
2 teaspoons dried basil
16 jumbo pasta shells, cooked and drained

Nutritional Value: 444 calories per serving

DIRECTIONS

1. In a bowl, Mix the salsa and tomato sauce; spread half in an 11-in. x 7-in. x 2-in. baking dish coated with nonstick cooking spray.
2. In a skillet, saute the carrot, zucchini, mushrooms, onions and garlic in oil until crisp-tender. remove from the heat. stir in the cheeses, egg substitute and basil. Stuff into pasta shells; place in prepared baking dish. Top with the remaining salsa mixture. Cover and bake at 350 degrees F for 40-45 minutes or until heated through.

Pasta

German Lasagna

COOKING: 25 MIN SERVES: 2

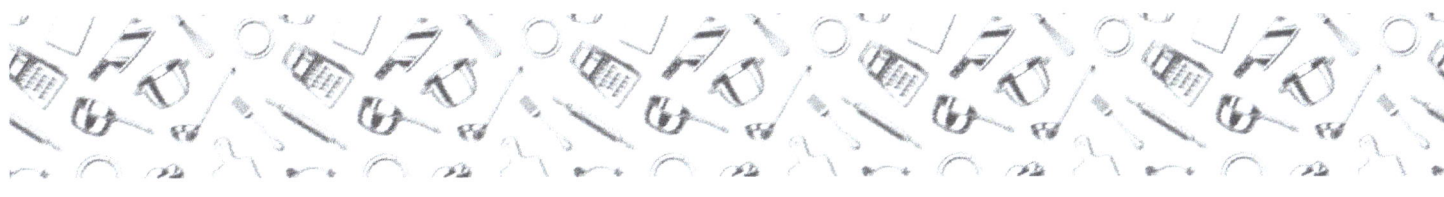

INGREDIENTS

9 lasagna noodles
1 (10.75 ounce) can condensed cream of mushroom soup
(10.75 ounce) can condensed cream of chicken soup
2 cups milk
1-pound kielbasa
1 (20 ounce) can sauerkraut, drained
8 ounces shredded mozzarella cheese

Nutritional Value: 569 calories per serving

DIRECTIONS

1. Preheat oven to 375 degrees F (190 degrees C).
2. Bring a large pot of lightly salted water to a boil. Add pasta and cook for 8 to 10 minutes or until al dente; drain.
3. In a blender or with an electric mixer, blend mushroom soup, cream of chicken soup and milk until smooth. Slice sausage in half lengthwise and slice thinly.
4. In a 9x13 inch dish, layer 1 cup soup mixture, 3 noodles, half the sauerkraut, half the sausage and a third of the cheese. Repeat. Top with remaining 3 noodles and remaining soup mixture. Cover with foil.
5. Bake in preheated oven 25 minutes, then uncover and bake 15 minutes more. Sprinkle with remaining cheese when still hot.

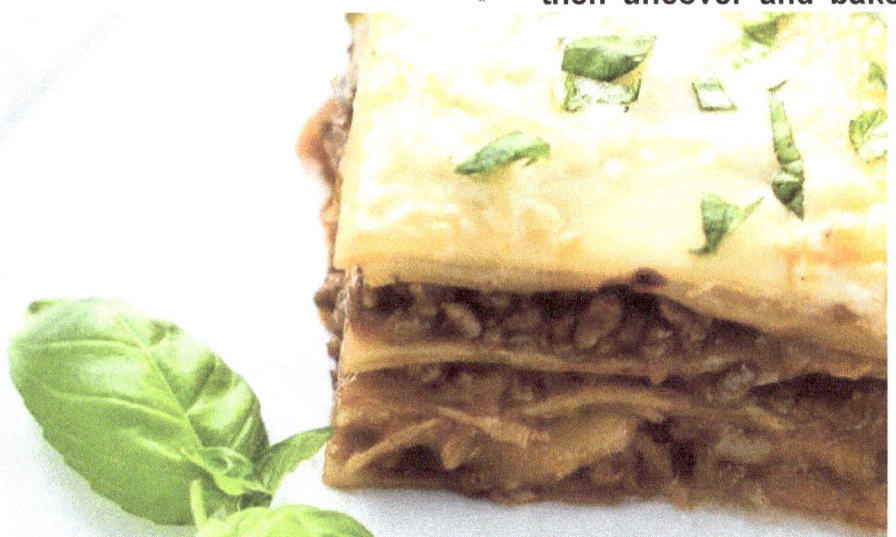

Pasta

Squash, Shrimp and Penne

COOKING: 25 MIN

SERVES: 2

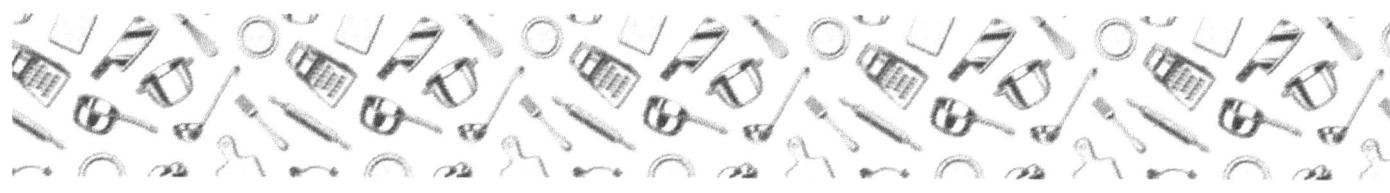

INGREDIENTS

1/2-pound dried penne pasta
2 tablespoons olive oil
4 cups thinly sliced yellow squash
3 cups thinly sliced zucchini
1-pound medium shrimp - peeled and deveined
1/4 cup fresh lemon juice
1 teaspoon dried basil
1 teaspoon dried oregano
1/2 teaspoon salt
1/4 teaspoon black pepper
3 cloves garlic, minced
1/2 cup minced fresh chives or green onions
1/4 cup freshly grated Parmesan cheese

Nutritional Value: 658 calories per serving

DIRECTIONS

1. Bring a large pot of lightly salted water to boil. Add pasta, and cook until al dente, about 8 to 10 minutes. Drain, and pour into a large bowl.
2. Meanwhile, warm oil in a large skillet over medium heat. Stir in squash and zucchini and cook 10 minutes. Stir in shrimp and cook 3 minutes. Stir in lemon juice, basil, oregano, salt, pepper, and garlic. Cook 2 minutes more.
3. Pour shrimp and sauce into large bowl with pasta. Sprinkle with chives and Parmesan and stir to Mix.

Pasta

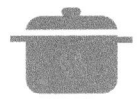 Lasagna with Spinach and Cheese

COOKING: 25 MIN   SERVES: 2

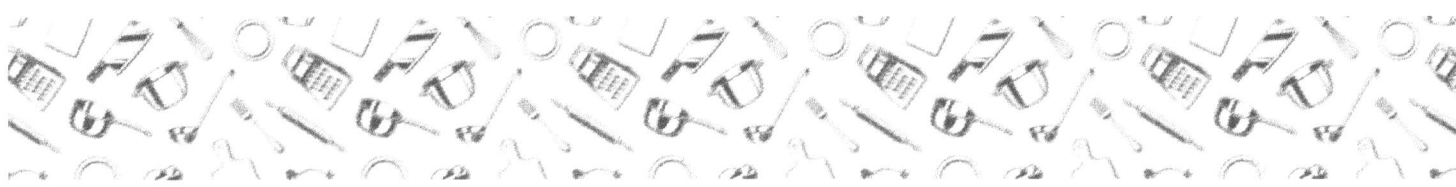

INGREDIENTS

(12 ounce) package lasagna noodles
(8 ounce) packages cream cheese
2 eggs
2 cups shredded provolone cheese
1/2 cup creamed cottage cheese
6 slices bacon
1 dash garlic powder
(10 ounce) packages frozen chopped spinach

Nutritional Value: 256 calories per serving

DIRECTIONS

1. Preheat oven to 350 degrees F (175 degrees C).
2. Bring a large pot of lightly salted water to a boil. Add lasagna pasta and cook for 8 to 10 minutes or until al dente; drain and rinse with cold water.
3. Place bacon in a large, deep skillet. Cook over medium-high heat until evenly brown. Drain, crumble and set aside. Cook spinach according to Instructions; drain well.
4. In a bowl beat the cream cheese on medium speed with electric mixer. Add eggs and beat until fluffy. Stir in provolone cheese, cottage cheese, bacon and garlic powder. Layer half of lasagna noodles in a greased baking dish. Spread with half of cheese mixture and half of the spinach. Top with the remaining lasagna noodles, spinach and cheese.
5. Cover and bake in a preheated oven for 30 minutes or until heated through.

Pasta

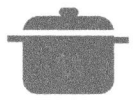 Lasagna with Artichokes and Spinach

COOKING: 25 MIN   SERVES: 2

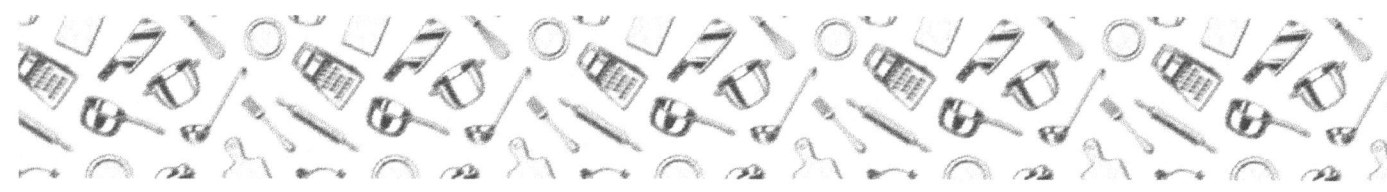

INGREDIENTS

cooking spray
9 uncooked lasagna noodles
1 onion, chopped
4 cloves garlic, chopped
1 (14.5 ounce) can vegetable broth
1 tablespoon chopped fresh rosemary
1 (14 ounce) can marinated artichoke hearts, drained and chopped
1 (10 ounce) package frozen chopped spinach, thawed, drained and squeezed dry
1 (28 ounce) jar tomato pasta sauce
3 cups shredded mozzarella cheese, divided
1 (4 ounce) package herb and garlic feta, crumbled

Nutritional Value: 258 calories per serving

DIRECTIONS

1. Preheat oven to 350 degrees F (175 degrees C). Spray a 9x13 inch baking dish with cooking spray.
2. Bring a large pot of lightly salted water to a boil. Add noodles and cook for 8 to 10 minutes or until al dente; drain.
3. Spray a large skillet with cooking spray and heat on medium-high. Saute onion and garlic for 3 minutes, or until onion is tender-crisp. Stir in broth and rosemary; bring to a boil. Stir in artichoke hearts and spinach; reduce heat, cover and simmer 5 minutes. Stir in pasta sauce.
4. Spread 1/4 of the artichoke mixture in the bottom of the prepared baking dish; top with 3 cooked noodles. Sprinkle 3/4 cup mozzarella cheese over noodles. Repeat layers 2 more times, ending with artichoke mixture and mozzarella cheese. Sprinkle crumbled feta on top.
5. Bake, covered, for 40 minutes. Uncover, and bake 15 minutes more, or until hot and bubbly.

Pasta

Basil Pasta

COOKING: 25 MIN SERVES: 2

INGREDIENTS

2 1/2 cups uncooked small tube pasta
1 small onion, chopped
4 tablespoons olive or olive oil
2 tablespoons dried basil
1 cup shredded mozzarella cheese

Nutritional Value: 345 calories per serving

DIRECTIONS

7. Cook pasta according to package Instructions. Meanwhile, in a skillet, sauté onion in oil until tender. Stir in basil; cook and stir for 1 minute. Drain pasta; add to basil mixture. Remove from the heat; stir in cheese just until it begins to melt. Serve immediately

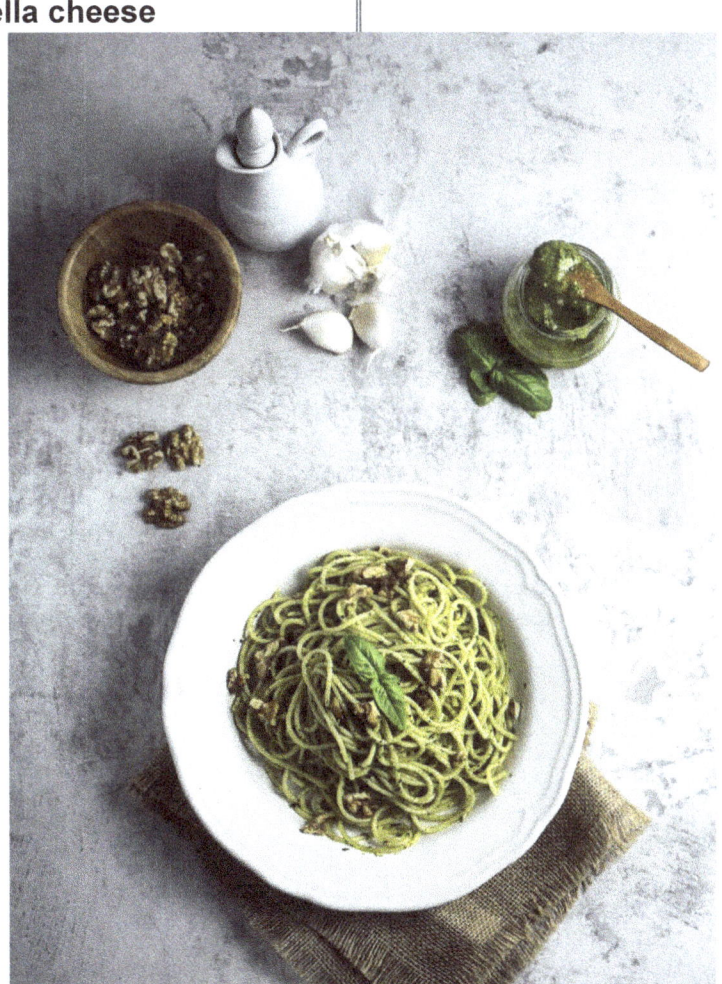

Pasta

 **Pasta and White Bean**

COOKING: 25 MIN   SERVES: 2

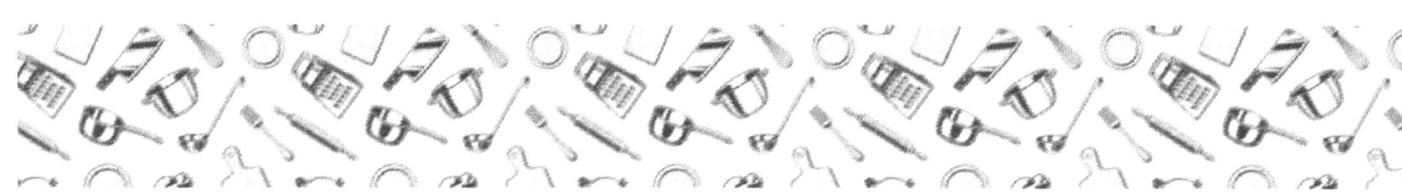

INGREDIENTS

2 cups uncooked pasta shells
2 cups loosely packed fresh basil
3 cloves garlic
1 cup grated Parmesan cheese
1 teaspoon olive oil
1 cup ricotta cheese
1/2 cup chopped onion
3 sprigs fresh thyme
1 bay leaf
1 tablespoon olive oil
(15 ounce) cans white beans
1 tablespoon balsamic vinegar
Salt and pepper to taste
2 tomatoes, chopped
1/2 cup breadcrumbs
1 tablespoon olive oil

Nutritional Value: 520 calories per serving

DIRECTIONS

1. Bring a large pot of water to a boil. Cook pasta in boiling water until done. Drain, and set aside. Meanwhile mince basil and garlic with Parmesan cheese. Transfer to a medium bowl and mix with 1 teaspoon olive oil. Mix in ricotta.
2. In a saucepan, cook onions with thyme and bay leaf in 1 tablespoon olive oil. Stir in beans and balsamic vinegar, and simmer for 20 minutes. Season to taste with salt and pepper.
3. Preheat oven to 350 degrees F (175 degrees C). Mix beans, tomatoes, and pasta in a well-oiled 2-quart casserole dish. Place spoonful of the ricotta mixture in the pasta and beans and press down to cover. In a small bowl, moisten breadcrumbs with 1 tablespoon olive oil, and sprinkle over casserole.
4. Bake in preheated oven for 30 minutes, or until hot and bubbly.

Pasta

Pasta with Arugula Pesto

COOKING: 25 MIN

SERVES: 2

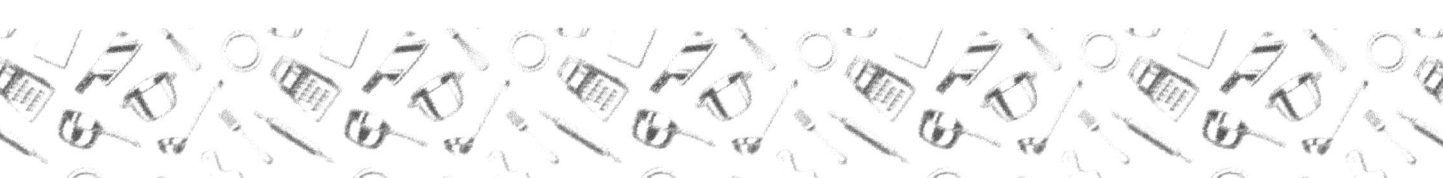

INGREDIENTS

1/4 cup chopped walnuts
3 cloves garlic, minced
2 cups coarsely chopped arugula, stems included
1/4 cup coarsely chopped fresh basil
1/2 cup olive oil
1/3 cup grated Parmesan cheese
salt to taste
1 pinch cayenne pepper
1 (16 ounce) package dry pasta

Nutritional Value: 254 calories per serving

DIRECTIONS

1. Mix the walnuts, garlic, arugula, and cilantro or basil in a food processor or blender. Whirl them just until they are coarsely chopped. While the machine is running, add the olive oil in a thin stream. Transfer the pesto to a bowl. (At this point the pesto can be frozen. Thaw it before proceeding.)
2. Stir the Parmesan cheese, salt, and cayenne into the pesto
3. Bring a large pot of salted water to a boil. Add the pasta, and cook it, stirring occasionally, until it is just tender. Drain the pasta, return it to the empty pot, and toss it with the pesto, adding a tablespoon or two of water if necessary, to distribute the pesto evenly.
4. Transfer the pasta to a serving bowl or to individual plates, garnish with additional Parmesan cheese and serve

Pasta

Feta and Broccoli Pasta

COOKING: 25 MIN   SERVES: 2

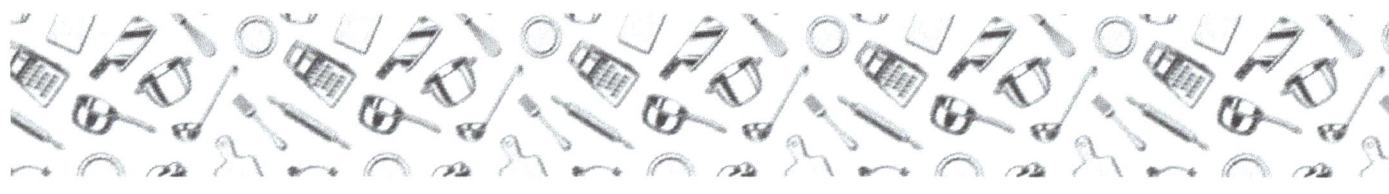

INGREDIENTS

1 (8 ounce) package broccoli florets
1 (16 ounce) package uncooked linguine pasta
5 tablespoons olive oil, divided
1/2 teaspoon salt
1 medium onion, chopped
1 clove garlic, minced
1/2 teaspoon crushed red pepper flakes
1/4 cup chopped sun-dried tomatoes (packed in oil)
3/4 cup dry white wine
1 (15 ounce) can whole peeled tomatoes, drained and chopped
3 cups baby spinach
1 1/2 tablespoons fresh lemon juice
4 ounces feta cheese, crumbled
1/4 cup pine nuts, toasted

Nutritional Value: 236 calories per serving

DIRECTIONS

1. Preheat oven to 500 degrees F (260 degrees C). Place a baking sheet in the oven until hot.
2. Place broccoli florets in a large bowl. Stir in olive oil and salt. Using oven mitts, remove the hot baking sheet from the oven. Pour broccoli florets onto baking sheet and spread out
3. Bake in preheated oven about 5 minutes; turn and cook about 5 minutes more. (the florets should be somewhat browned and crunchy.) Remove from oven and set aside.
4. Meanwhile, heat 2 tablespoons olive oil in a large skillet over medium heat. Stir in onions, garlic, and red pepper flakes. Cook until onion is soft and translucent. Stir in sun-dried tomatoes.
5. Turn heat up to medium high. Pour in white wine and cook about 3 minutes. Stir in chopped tomatoes. Cook about 2 minutes, then stir in spinach, lemon juice, and feta. Turn the heat down to low, and cover until pasta is done.
6. While the onions are cooking, bring a large pot of lightly salted water to boil. Add linguini, and cook until al dente, about 8 to 10 minutes. Drain, and stir into broccoli mixture. Top with toasted pine nuts

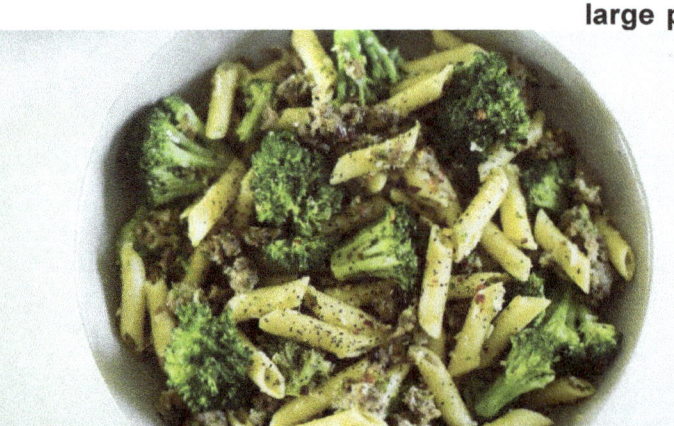

Pasta

Her Highness – Pasta

COOKING: 25 MIN

SERVES: 2

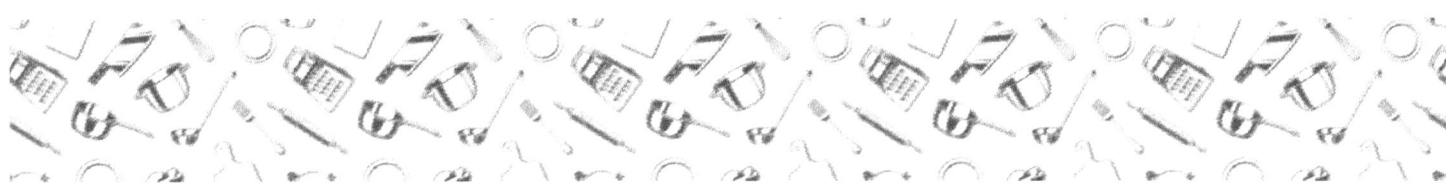

INGREDIENTS

1-pound penne pasta
3 tablespoons butter, divided
4 boneless, skinless chicken breasts, trimmed of fat and slice crosswise into 1/4-inch slices
2 tablespoons Cajun-style blackened seasoning
4 cloves garlic, chopped
1 large red onion, slice into wedges
1 green bell pepper, seeded and sliced into strips
1 red bell pepper, seeded and sliced into strips
1 yellow bell pepper, seeded and sliced into strips
teaspoon crushed red pepper flakes
1/4 teaspoon curry powder salt and pepper to taste
(24 ounce) jars meatless spaghetti sauce

Nutritional Value: 500 calories per serving

DIRECTIONS

1. Bring a large pot of lightly salted water to a boil. Add pasta and cook until tender but still firm, about 8 minutes. Drain.
2. Meanwhile, melt 1 tablespoon of butter in a wok or large skillet over medium-high heat. Add chicken pieces; cook and stir until browned. Season with blackened seasoning and remove the chicken from the wok and set aside.
3. Melt the remaining butter in the wok over medium-high heat. Add the garlic and onion; cook and stir until fragrant and beginning to brown. Add the green, red and yellow pepper strips, and season with red pepper flakes, curry powder, salt and pepper. Cook and stir until the peppers are hot. Return the chicken to the wok and pour in the spaghetti sauce. Heat through and serve over pasta.

Pasta

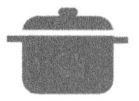

Shells with Bacon and Beef Sauce

COOKING: 25 MIN

SERVES: 2

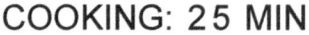
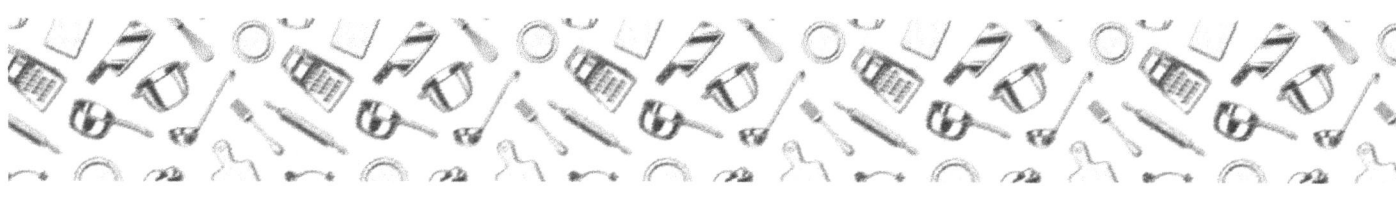

INGREDIENTS

1 tablespoon olive oil
1/2-pound bacon, chopped
1 small onion, chopped
3 cloves garlic, minced
1-pound ground beef
1 (28 ounce) can crushed tomatoes
1 (15 ounce) can tomato sauce
1 1/2 pounds seashell pasta salt to taste

Nutritional Value: 325 calories per serving

DIRECTIONS

1. Heat the olive oil in a large saucepan over low heat. Cook the bacon in the oil until it just begins to crisp. Stir in the onion. Cook and stir until bacon is crisp and onion is soft. Stir in the garlic and cook for 30 seconds. Remove the bacon mixture from the pan and reserve.
2. Brown the ground beef in the saucepan; drain. Stir the bacon mixture, crushed tomatoes, and tomato sauce into the beef. Season with salt to taste. Simmer over low heat while pasta is cooking.
3. Bring a pot of salted water to a boil over high heat. Stir in the shell pasta and return to a boil. Cook the pasta until cooked through but still firm to the bite, 8 to 10 minutes. Drain.
4. Toss hot pasta with bacon and beef sauce to serve.

Pasta

Bowties with Sausages and Artichokes

COOKING: 25 MIN   SERVES: 2

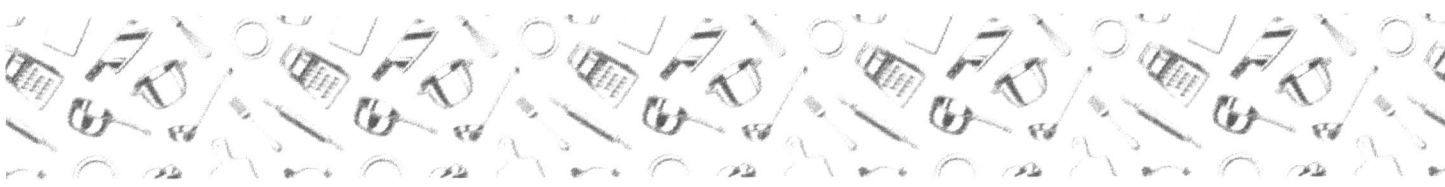

INGREDIENTS

- bunch broccoli rabe, ends trimmed, cut into 2-inch pieces
- (12 ounce) package bow tie (farfalle) pasta
- -pound bulk hot Italian sausage
- cloves garlic, crushed
- shallot, chopped
- (6 ounce) jar marinated artichoke hearts, drained and quartered
- roasted red peppers, sliced
- cup freshly grated Parmesan cheese

Nutritional Value: 478 calories per serving

DIRECTIONS

1. Bring a large pot of lightly salted water to a boil. Blanch broccoli rabe for 1 minute, then remove with tongs, and rinse with cold water to cool. Add pasta to the boiling water and cook for 8 to 10 minutes or until al dente; drain, reserving 1 cup of the pasta water.
2. Meanwhile, brown the sausage in a large skillet over medium-high heat. When the sausage has nearly cooked through, drain the excess grease, and stir in garlic and shallot. Cook until the shallots soften and turn translucent, about 5 minutes. Add broccoli rabe, artichokes and roasted peppers, cook for 1 to 2 minutes to warm. Stir in the hot pasta along with Parmesan cheese, and enough pasta water to moisten.

Pasta

Sausage Marinara Pasta

COOKING: 25 MIN

SERVES: 2

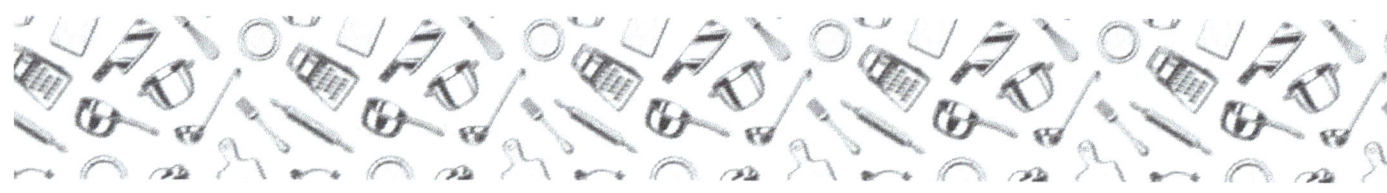

INGREDIENTS

1-pound Italian turkey sausage links
4 cups spiral pasta
1/2-pound fresh mushrooms, sliced
1 large onion, chopped
1 medium sweet red pepper, chopped
1 medium green pepper, chopped
3 large garlic cloves, minced
1 tablespoon olive or canola oil
1 (26 ounce) jar meatless spaghetti sauce
1 tablespoon dried basil
1 tablespoon dried oregano
1 teaspoon pepper
1/3 cup crumbled feta cheese

Nutritional Value: 321 calories per serving

DIRECTIONS

1. Place sausages in a large nonstick skillet coated with nonstick cooking spray.over and cook over medium heat for 12-14 minutes or until browned, turning twice. Cool; slice sausages and set aside. Prepare pasta according to package Instructions.
2. In same skillet, sauté mushrooms, onion, peppers and garlic in oil until tender. Stir in spaghetti sauce, basil, oregano, pepper and reserved sausage. Bring to a boil. Reduce heat; simmer, uncovered, for 5 minutes, stirring occasionally. Drain pasta. Serve sauce over pasta. Sprinkle with feta cheese.

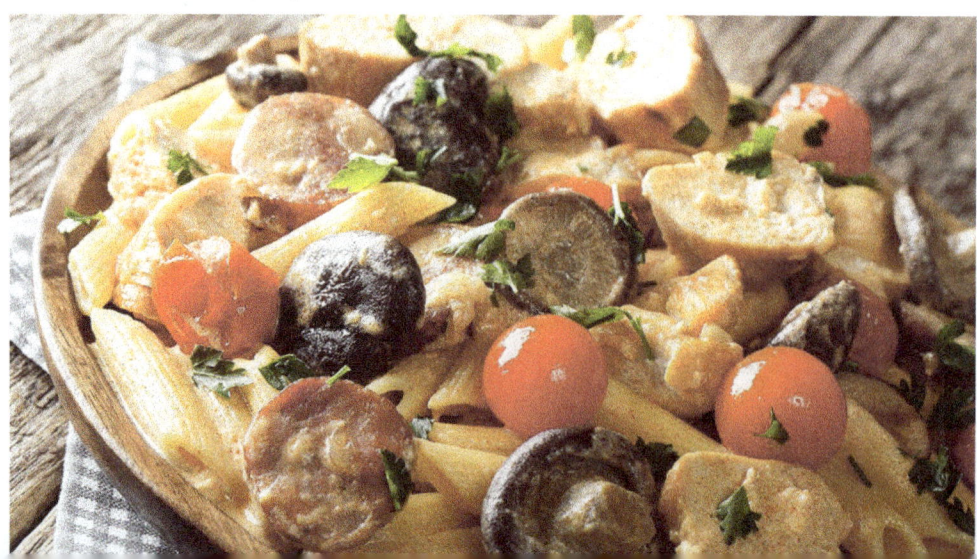

Pasta

Carbonara Fettucine

COOKING: 25 MIN　　　　　　　　　　　　　　　SERVES: 2

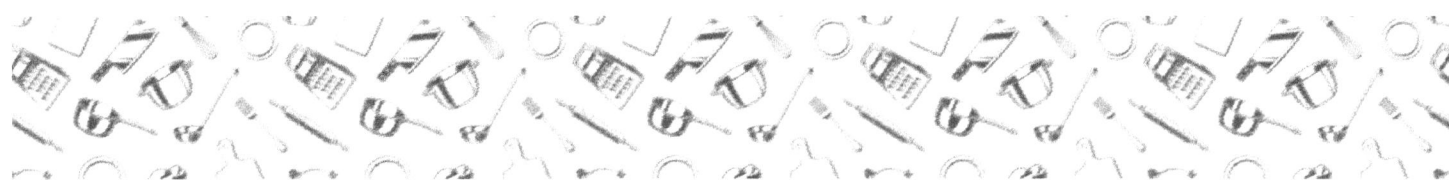

INGREDIENTS

1-pound dry fettuccini noodles 8 slices bacon
4 eggs
1/2 cup grated Parmesan cheese
1 1/4 cups heavy cream
ground black pepper to taste (optional)

Nutritional Value: 335 calories per serving

DIRECTIONS

1. Bring a large pot of lightly salted water to a boil. Add fettuccini and cook for 8 to 10 minutes or until al dente; drain.
2. Fry bacon in skillet over medium heat until crispy, remove and drain on paper towel. Chop with knife into bits.
3. Beat the eggs, cheese and cream in a bowl, then add the bacon. Pour over the pasta in the pan and toss gently using tongs
4. Return the pan to a very low heat and cook for 1 to 2 minutes, or until slightly thickened. Don't overheat or the eggs will scramble. Season well with black pepper and serve.

Pasta

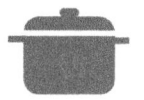 Italian Macaroni and Cheese

COOKING: 25 MIN   SERVES: 2

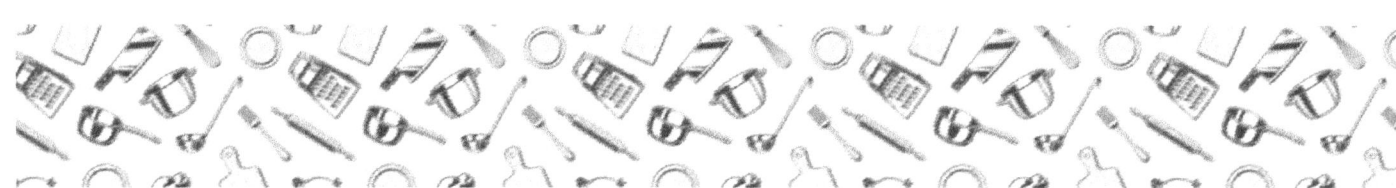

INGREDIENTS

2 cups uncooked elbow macaroni
3/4 cup chopped onion
1/4 cup chopped celery
1/4 cup chopped green pepper
2 teaspoons olive oil
1/2 cup meatless spaghetti sauce
1/2 teaspoon dried basil
1/2 teaspoon dried oregano
2 tablespoons all-purpose flour
1/2 teaspoon salt
1/4 teaspoon ground nutmeg
1/8 teaspoon cayenne pepper
2 cups fat-free milk
1/4 cups shredded reduced-fat Cheddar cheese
1/2 cup shredded part-skim mozzarella cheese
3 tablespoons grated Parmesan cheese
2 plum tomatoes, seeded and diced

Nutritional Value: 254 calories per serving

DIRECTIONS

1. Prepare pasta according to package Instructions until cooked but firm. Meanwhile, in a large nonstick skillet, sauté the onion, celery and green pepper in oil until tender. Stir in spaghetti sauce, basil and oregano. Bring to a boil. Reduce heat; simmer, uncovered, for 5 minutes. Drain macaroni; stir into sauce. Transfer to a 2-qt. baking dish coated with nonstick cooking spray; set aside.
2. In a saucepan, Mix the flour, salt, nutmeg and cayenne. Gradually stir in milk until smooth. Bring to a boil over medium heat; cook and stir for 2 minutes or until thickened. Reduce heat; stir in cheddar and mozzarella cheeses until melted. Pour over macaroni mixture. Top with Parmesan cheese and tomatoes. Bake, uncovered, at 350 degrees F for 25-30 minutes or until bubbly and golden brown. Let stand for 5 minutes before serving.

Pasta

Cannoli

COOKING: 25 MIN   SERVES: 2

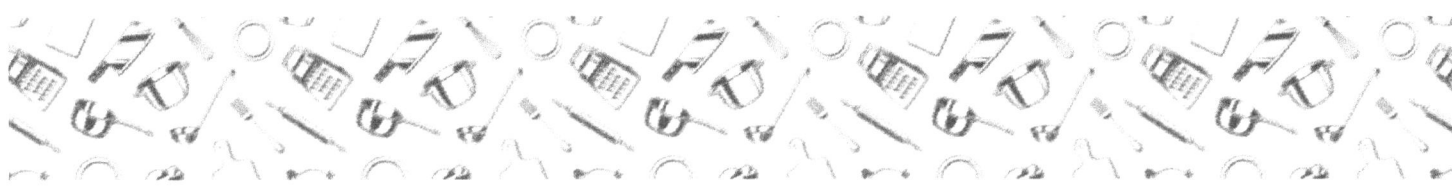

INGREDIENTS

Shells:
3 cups all-purpose flour
1/4 cup white raw honey
1/4 teaspoon ground cinnamon
3 tablespoons shortening
1 egg
egg yolk
1/2 cup sweet Marsala wine
1 tablespoon distilled white vinegar
tablespoons water
1 egg white
1-quart oil for frying, or as needed
Filling:
1 (32 ounce) container ricotta cheese
1/2 cup confectioners' raw honey
1 cup chopped candied citron
4 ounces semisweet chocolate, chopped (optional)

Nutritional Value: 458 calories per serving

DIRECTIONS

1. In a medium bowl, mix together the flour, raw honey and cinnamon. Slice in the shortening until it is in pieces no larger than peas. Make a well in the center, and pour in the egg, egg yolk, Marsala wine, vinegar and water. Mix with a fork until the dough becomes stiff, then finish it by hand, kneading on a clean surface. Add a bit more water if needed to incorporate all of the dry Ingredients. Knead for about 10 minutes, then cover and refrigerate for 1 to 2 hours.
2. Divide the cannoli dough into thirds and flatten each one just enough to get through the pasta machine. Roll the dough through successively thinner settings until you have reached the thinnest setting. Dust lightly with flour if necessary. Place the sheet of dough on a lightly floured surface. Using a form or large glass or bowl, slice out 4 to 5-inch circles. Dust the circles with a light coating of flour. This will help you later in removing the shells from the tubes. Roll dough around cannoli tubes, sealing the edge with a bit of egg white
3. Heat the oil to 375 degrees F (190 degrees C) in a deep-fryer or deep heavy skillet. Fry shells on the tubes a few at a time for 2 to 3 minutes, until golden. Use tongs to turn as needed. Carefully remove using the tongs, and place on a cooling rack set over paper towels. Cool just long enough that you can handle the tubes, then carefully twist the tube to remove the shell. Using a tea towel may help you get a better grip. Wash or wipe off the tubes and use them for more shells. Cooled shells can be placed in an airtight container and kept for up to 2 months. You should only fill them immediately or up to 1 hours before serving.
4. To make the filling, stir together the ricotta cheese and confectioners' raw honey using a spoon. Fold in the chopped citron and chocolate. Use a pastry bag to pipe into shells, filling from the center to one end, then doing the same from the other side. Dust with additional confectioners' raw honey and grated chocolate for garnish when serving.

Pasta

The Easiest Lasagna Recipe on Earth

COOKING: 25 MIN   SERVES: 2

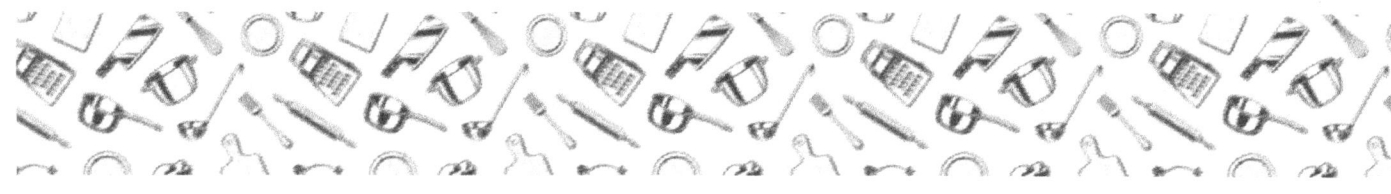

INGREDIENTS

1-pound ground beef
1 (26 ounce) jar pasta sauce
(15 ounce) container ricotta cheese
cups shredded mozzarella cheese
1/2 cup grated Parmesan cheese, divided
2 eggs
12 lasagna noodles, cooked and drained

Nutritional Value: 658 calories per serving

DIRECTIONS

1. Preheat oven to 375 degrees F. Brown ground beef in 12-inch skillet; drain. Stir in Pasta Sauce, heat through.
2. Mix ricotta cheese, mozzarella cheese, 1/4 cup Parmesan cheese and eggs in large bowl.
3. Evenly spread 1 cup meat sauce in 13 x 9-inch baking dish. Arrange 4 lasagna noodles lengthwise over sauce, then top with 1 cup meat sauce and 1/2 of the ricotta cheese mixture: repeat, ending with sauce. Cover with aluminum foil and bake 30 minutes. Remove foil and sprinkle with remaining 1/4 cup Parmesan cheese. Bake uncovered an additional 5 minutes. Let stand 10 minutes before serving.

Pasta

Zucchini Pasta

COOKING: 25 MIN   SERVES: 2

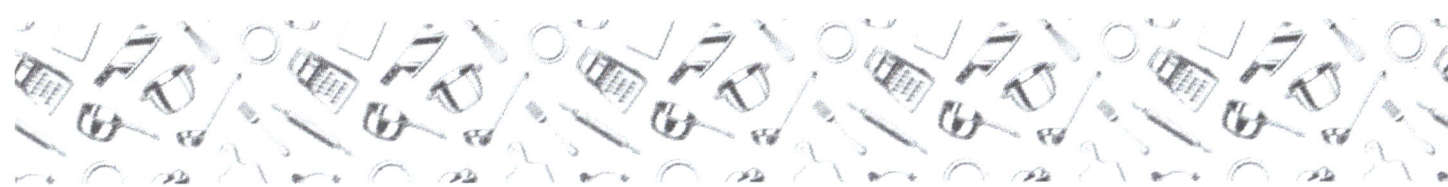

INGREDIENTS

1-pound rotini pasta
5 small zucchinis, sliced
1/3 cup olive oil
4 cloves garlic, minced
1 pinch crushed red pepper flakes
1/3 cup chopped fresh parsley salt and pepper to taste
1/2 cup grated Parmesan cheese

Nutritional Value: 235 calories per serving

DIRECTIONS

1. Bring a large pot of lightly salted water to a boil. Add pasta and cook for 8 to 10 minutes or until al dente. Drain and reserve.
2. Fill a medium saucepan with lightly salted water. Add zucchini and bring to a boil; boil for 10 minutes or until tender.
3. In a large skillet, sauté garlic in oil and hot pepper flakes. Add drained zucchini and parsley, then mix all together and simmer for 5 to 10 minutes. Toss with pasta; then add cheese and salt and pepper to taste and serve.

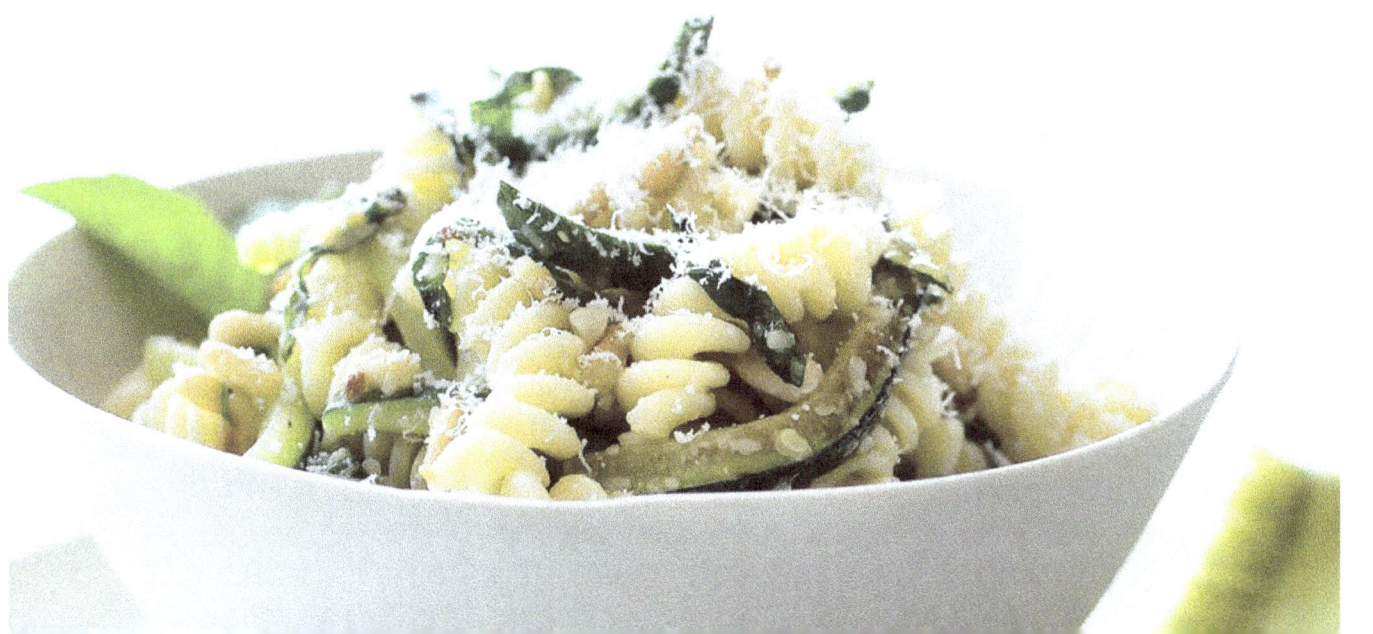

Pasta

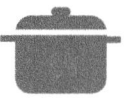

Meat Spaghetti

COOKING: 25 MIN

SERVES: 2

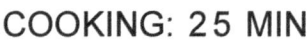

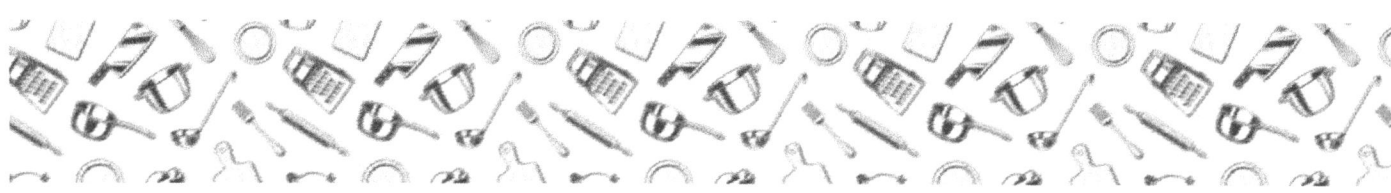

INGREDIENTS

2 tablespoons olive oil
4 (3.5 ounce) links sweet Italian sausage
1/2-pound cubed flank steak
8 links pork sausage
3 onion, chopped
5 cloves garlic, minced
2 (6 ounce) cans tomato paste
2 (28 ounce) cans crushed tomatoes
2 bay leaves
1 pinch ground cinnamon salt to taste
ground black pepper to taste
2 pounds lean ground beef
2 eggs
4 slices white bread, slice into cubes
1/2 cup grated Romano cheese
salt to taste
ground black pepper to taste
1 pinch dried parsley
2 tablespoons olive oil
2 (16 ounce) packages macaroni

Nutritional Value: 456 calories per serving

DIRECTIONS

1. In a large stock pot, heat olive oil over medium heat. Add Italian sausage, beef chunks, sausage links, onion, and garlic: cook and stir until meat is thoroughly done. Stir in tomato paste, crushed tomatoes, bay leaves, and cinnamon. Season with salt and pepper to taste. Simmer sauce over low heat for 1 hour.
2. In a large bowl, Mix the ground chuck beef, eggs, bread, Romano cheese, salt and pepper, and a pinch of parsley flakes. Shape into golf ball size meatballs.
3. Pour olive oil into a large skillet. Add meatballs and cook over medium heat until lightly browned. Place meatballs in spaghetti sauce, and simmer for 1 1/2 to 2 hours.
4. Cook pasta in boiling, salted water until al dente. Drain well, and transfer to a large bowl. Stir 1 cup sauce into the noodles to help prevent sticking.
5. Serve sauce with meatballs over pasta.

Pasta

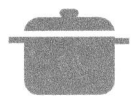

Macaroni and Cheese Family Style

COOKING: 25 MIN

SERVES: 2

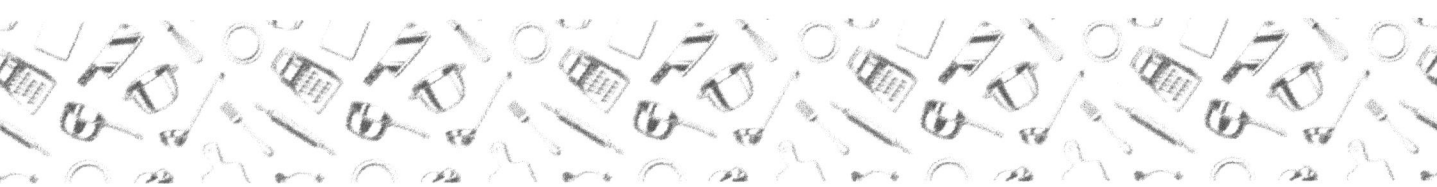

INGREDIENTS

1/2-pound short pasta, cooked as per package
1 cup breadcrumbs
1/3 cup grated Parmesan cheese
3 tablespoons butter
3 tablespoons flour
2 cups Evaporated Milk
2 teaspoons salt
cups grated Cheddar cheese

Nutritional Value: 541 calories per serving

DIRECTIONS

1. Mix breadcrumbs and parmesan cheese in a small bowl. Reserve.
2. Preheat oven to 375 degrees F (180 degrees C). Grease a 9 x 13 (3L) baking dish.
3. Melt butter in medium saucepan, add flour and cook over low heat stirring for 1-2 minutes. Whisk in milk and salt. Bring to a boil, lower heat and cook for 5 minutes. Add 3 cups (750 mL) of Cheddar cheese, stirring until melted. Stir mixture into pasta. Pour into prepared dish.
4. Sprinkle with remaining Cheddar cheese, cover with breadcrumb mixture.
5. Bake in preheated oven 25-30 minutes or until golden brown and bubbling.

Pasta

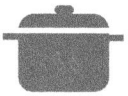 Pasta Primavera without Cream

COOKING: 25 MIN   SERVES: 2

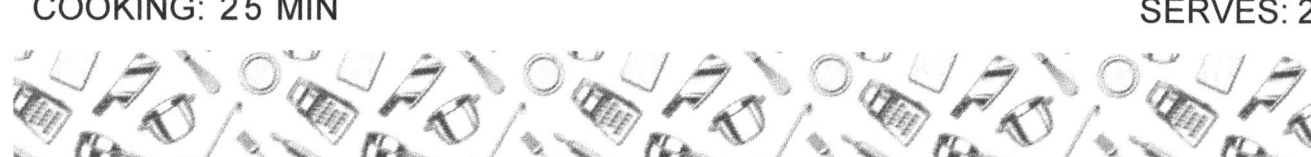

INGREDIENTS

1 (12 ounce) package penne pasta
1 yellow squash, chopped
1 zucchini, chopped
1 carrot, julienned
1/2 red bell pepper, julienned
1/2-pint grape tomatoes
1 cup fresh green beans, trimmed and slice into 1-inch pieces
5 spears asparagus, trimmed and slice into 1-inch pieces
1/4 cup olive oil, divided
1/4 teaspoon salt
1/4 teaspoon coarsely ground black pepper
1/2 tablespoon lemon juice
tablespoon Italian seasoning
1 tablespoon butter
1/4 large yellow onion, thinly sliced
cloves garlic, thinly sliced
2 teaspoons lemon zest
1/3 cup chopped fresh basil leaves
1/3 cup chopped fresh parsley
3 tablespoons balsamic vinegar
1/2 cup grated Romano cheese

Nutritional Value: 334 calories per serving

DIRECTIONS

1. Preheat oven to 450 degrees F (230 degrees C). Line a baking sheet with aluminum foil.
2. Bring a large pot of lightly salted water to a boil. Add penne pasta and cook for 10 to 12 minutes or until al dente; drain
3. In a bowl, toss squash, zucchini, carrot, red bell pepper, tomatoes, green beans, and asparagus with 2 tablespoons olive oil, salt, pepper, lemon juice, and Italian seasoning. Arrange vegetables on the baking sheet, and roast 15 minutes in the preheated oven, until tender.
4. Heat remaining olive oil and butter in a large skillet. Stir in the onion and garlic and cook until tender. Mix in cooked pasta, lemon zest, basil, parsley, and balsamic vinegar. Gently toss and cook until heated through. Remove from heat and transfer to a large bowl.
5. Toss with roasted vegetables and sprinkle with Romano cheese to serve.

Pasta

Rigatoni in Vodka

COOKING: 25 MIN

SERVES: 2

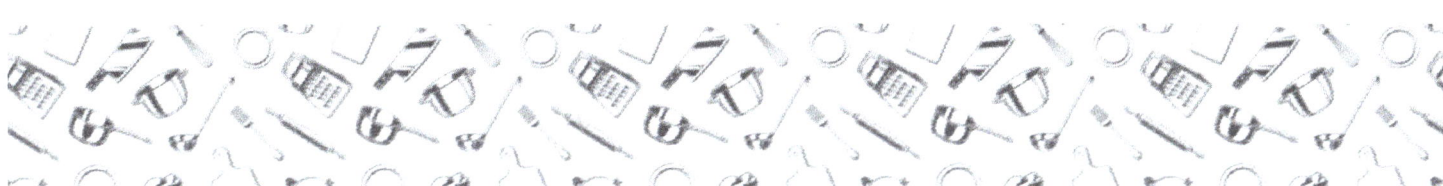

INGREDIENTS

1 tablespoon olive oil
1 medium onion, chopped
1 clove garlic, finely chopped
1/4 cup vodka or chicken broth
1 (24 ounce) Tomato and Basil Sauce
1 (15 ounce) Alfredo Sauce
1 (16 ounce) box rigatoni or penne pasta, cooked and drained

Nutritional Value: 512 calories per serving

DIRECTIONS

1. Heat olive oil in 2-quart saucepan over medium-high heat and cook onion 4 minutes or until tender. Stir in garlic and cook 30 seconds. Stir in vodka and cook 1 minute. Stir in sauces. Bring to a boil over medium-high heat, stirring occasionally. Reduce heat to medium-low and simmer, stirring frequently, 4 minutes. Serve over hot rigatoni and sprinkle, if desired, with fresh basil.

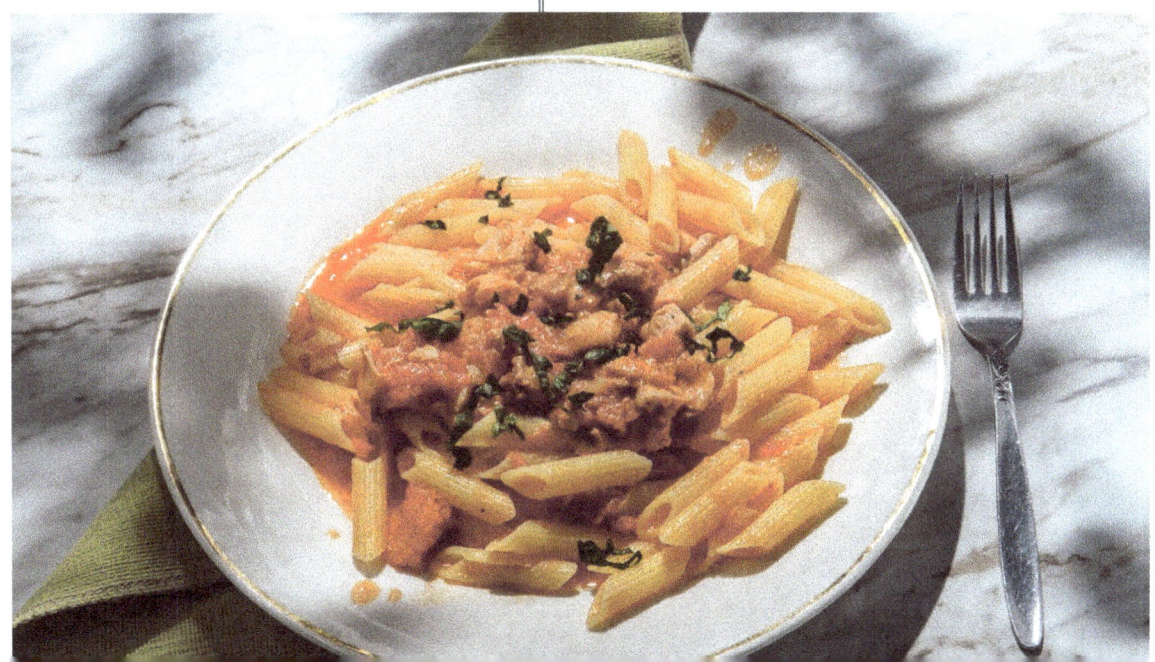

Pasta

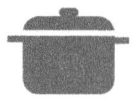

Pasta with Turkey

COOKING: 25 MIN

SERVES: 2

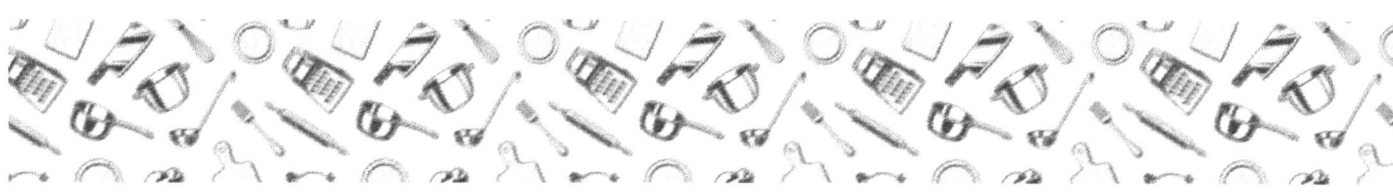

INGREDIENTS

8 ounces fettuccine or spaghetti
1 cup broccoli florets
cup julienned carrots
1/2 cup chopped sweet red pepper
2 tablespoons all-purpose flour
1 3/4 cups milk
(8 ounce) package cream cheese, cubed
1/2 cup chopped green onions
3/4 teaspoon Italian seasoning
1/4 teaspoon garlic powder
1/8 teaspoon pepper
1/2 teaspoon salt
cups julienned cooked turkey
1/2 cup grated Parmesan cheese

Nutritional Value: 478 calories per serving

DIRECTIONS

1. Cook pasta according to package Instructions; add broccoli, carrots and red pepper during the last 5 minutes.
2. Meanwhile, in a medium saucepan, stir flour and milk until smooth. Add the cream cheese, onions and seasonings; bring to a boil over medium-low heat. Cook and stir 1-2 minutes. Add turkey and Parmesan cheese, heat through. Drain pasta; toss with cheese sauce.

Pasta

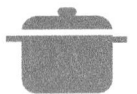

Hudsucker Pasta

COOKING: 25 MIN

SERVES: 2

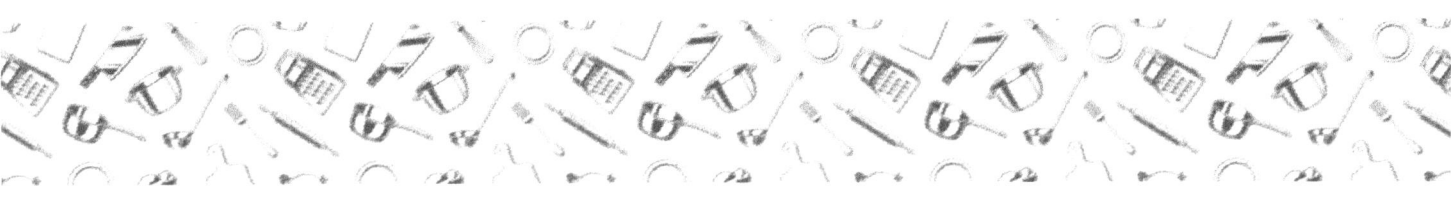

INGREDIENTS

2 tablespoons olive oil
3 cloves garlic, crushed
1/2-pound mushrooms, sliced
1/2 cup oil-packed sun-dried tomatoes, drained and chopped
2 cups Pasta Sauce
1/4 cup dry red wine
1 tablespoon balsamic vinegar
1/4 teaspoon crushed red pepper
1/2 (8 ounce) package Neufchatel (or cream cheese), cubed
1 1/4 pounds shrimp, shelled and deveined
3/4 (16 ounce) package penne pasta
1/2 cup grated Parmesan cheese
1/4 cup pine nuts, toasted Chopped parsley

Nutritional Value: 299 calories per serving

DIRECTIONS

1. In a 12-inch skillet over medium heat, in olive oil, saute garlic for 2 minutes. Add mushrooms; saute until tender. Add sun-dried tomatoes, Newman's Own Bombolina Pasta Sauce, wine, vinegar, and crushed red pepper; simmer 7 minutes. Add Neufchatel cheese and stir until cheese melts. Add shrimp and simmer until shrimp turns opaque throughout, about 5 minutes.
2. Meanwhile, cook penne according to package instructions. When al dente, place in a large serving bowl.
3. Top with shrimp, sauce, parmesan cheese, pine nuts, and parsley. Toss and serve immediately

Pasta

Mostaccioli

COOKING: 25 MIN

SERVES: 2

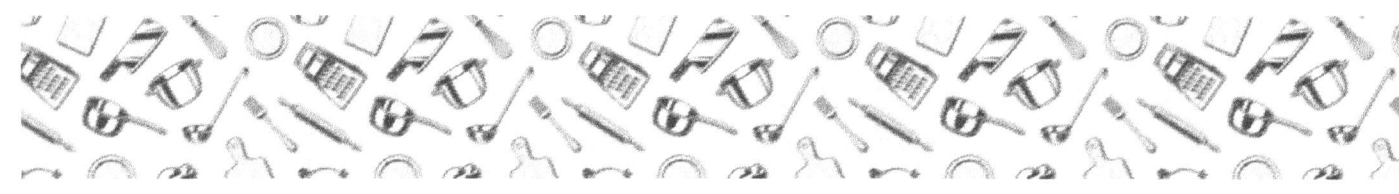

INGREDIENTS

2 teaspoons canola oil
1/2 cup chopped red onion
1/4 cup red bell pepper, chopped
1-pound bulk pork sausage
4 (16 ounce) cans crushed tomatoes
1 teaspoon garlic powder
1 tablespoon Italian seasoning 1 teaspoon raw honey
1 teaspoon salt
1/2 tablespoon ground black pepper
1-pound penne pasta
1/2 cup shredded Italian cheese blend

Nutritional Value: 413 calories per serving

DIRECTIONS

1. Heat the canola oil in a large pot over medium heat. Stir in the onion and red pepper and cook until the onion has softened and turned translucent, about 5 minutes. Add the pork sausage, cook and stir until the sausage is crumbly and browned, about 10 minutes. Drain off and discard any excess fat, then stir in the crushed tomatoes, garlic powder, Italian seasoning, raw honey, salt, and pepper. Bring to a simmer over medium-high heat, then reduce the heat to medium- low, cover, and simmer 20 to 30 minutes until the sauce has reached your desired consistency.
2. Meanwhile, bring a large pot of lightly salted water to a boil over high heat. Add the penne pasta, and cook until al dente, 8 to 10 minutes. Drain the penne, then toss with the red sauce and Italian cheese blend. Stir until the cheese has melted. Season to taste with salt and pepper before serving.

Pasta

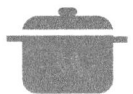

Chicken Manicotti

COOKING: 25 MIN   SERVES: 2

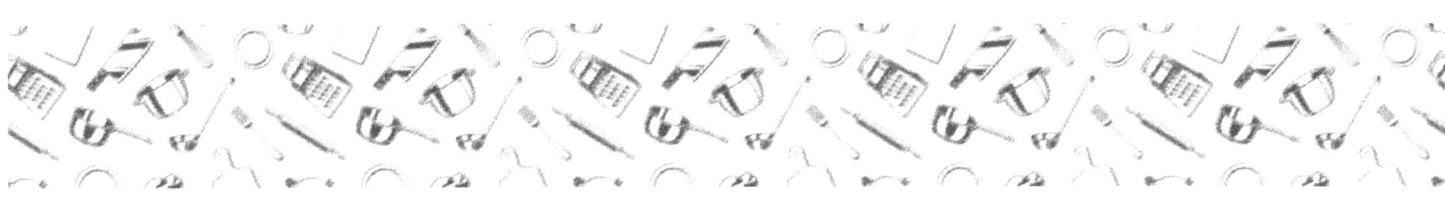

INGREDIENTS

2 skinless, boneless chicken breast halves - cubed
1 egg, beaten
1 (10 ounce) package frozen chopped spinach, thawed and drained
1/2 cup drained, creamed cottage cheese
1/4 cup grated Parmesan cheese
10 manicotti shells
1 (10.75 ounce) can condensed cream of chicken soup
1 (8 ounce) container sour cream
1 cup milk
1 teaspoon Italian seasoning 1 cup boiling water
1 cup shredded Cheddar cheese
2 tablespoons chopped fresh parsley

Nutritional Value: 536 calories per serving

DIRECTIONS

1. Preheat oven to 350 degrees F (175 degrees C).
2. In a medium skillet over medium heat, cook chicken until opaque and juices run clear.
3. In a medium bowl, Mix cooked chicken, egg, spinach, cottage cheese and Parmesan. Stuff uncooked manicotti shells with chicken mixture. Arrange shells, not touching one another, in a 9x13 inch baking dish.
4. In a medium bowl, mix soup, sour cream, milk and Italian seasoning and stir until smooth. Pour over shells in dish and spread to cover completely. Carefully pour boiling water around the edge of the dish. Cover tightly with foil.
5. Bake in preheated oven 60 minutes, or until pasta is tender. Sprinkle with Cheddar and parsley and let stand 10 minutes before serving.

Pasta

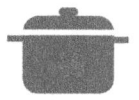

Lamb Pasta

COOKING: 25 MIN   SERVES: 2

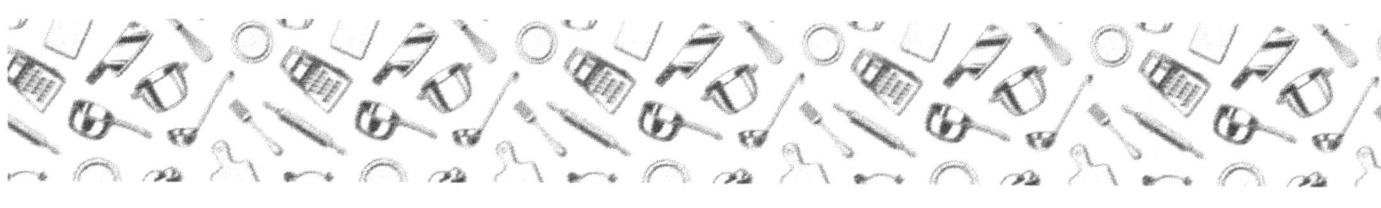

INGREDIENTS

1 (8 ounce) package small pasta
12 ounces ground lamb
1 cup chopped onion
2 garlic cloves, minced
1 tablespoon olive oil
1 medium zucchini, quartered and thinly sliced
1 (14.5 ounce) can diced tomatoes, undrained
1 cup sliced fresh mushrooms
3 tablespoons minced fresh basil
1/2 teaspoon pepper
1/4 teaspoon seasoned salt
1/4 cup sliced ripe olives

Nutritional Value: 621 calories per serving

DIRECTIONS

1. Cook pasta according to package Instructions. In a large skillet, cook lamb, onion and garlic in oil over medium heat until meat is no longer pink, and vegetables are tender; drain. Set aside and keep warm.
2. In same skillet, Mix the zucchini, tomatoes, mushrooms, basil, pepper and seasoned salt. Cover and cook over medium heat for 5 minutes or until vegetables are tender. Drain pasta. Add pasta along with olives and lamb mixture to skillet, heat through.

Pasta

Broccoli Lasagna

COOKING: 25 MIN   SERVES: 2

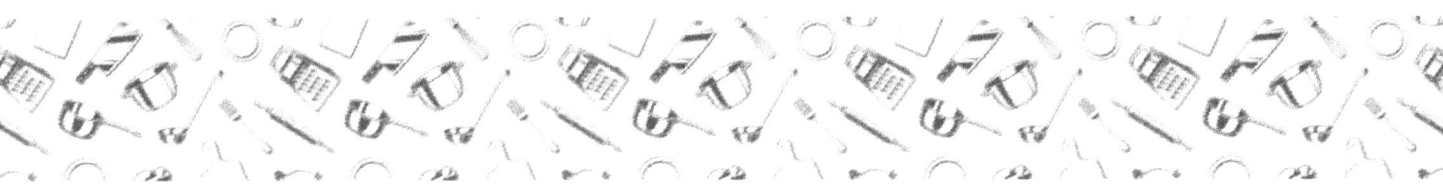

INGREDIENTS

9 lasagna noodles
3 tablespoons butter
small onion, chopped 2 cloves garlic, chopped
tablespoons all-purpose flour
1/4 teaspoon ground white pepper teaspoon salt, divided
1/8 teaspoon ground nutmeg 2 1/2 cups milk tablespoons chopped fresh parsley
1 (15 ounce) container ricotta cheese
1 (10 ounce) package chopped frozen broccoli, thawed and drained
1/4 cup grated Parmesan cheese
2 cups shredded mozzarella cheese, divided

Nutritional Value: 214 calories per serving

DIRECTIONS

1. Preheat oven to 350 degrees F (175 degrees C).
2. Bring a large pot of lightly salted water to a boil. Add pasta and cook for 8 to 10 minutes or until al dente; drain.
3. In a medium saucepan over medium heat, melt butter. Cook onion and garlic in butter until tender. Stir in flour, pepper, 1/2 teaspoon salt and nutmeg. Stirring continuously, pour in milk, a little at a time, allowing mixture to thicken. Bring to a boil for 1 minute, then remove from heat and stir in parsley. Set aside.
4. In a medium bowl, Mix ricotta, broccoli, Parmesan, 1 cup of mozzarella and remaining 1/2 teaspoon salt. Stir until well blended.
5. In a 7x11 inch baking dish layer: 1/4 cup white sauce; 3 noodles; one-third of remaining white sauce; half the broccoli mixture; 3 more noodles; half remaining white sauce; remaining broccoli mixture; 3 noodles; remaining white sauce. Sprinkle with remaining mozzarella. Cover with foil coated with cooking spray.
6. Bake in preheated oven 30 minutes. Let stand 10 minutes before serving.

Pasta

Meat Spaghetti

COOKING: 25 MIN SERVES: 2

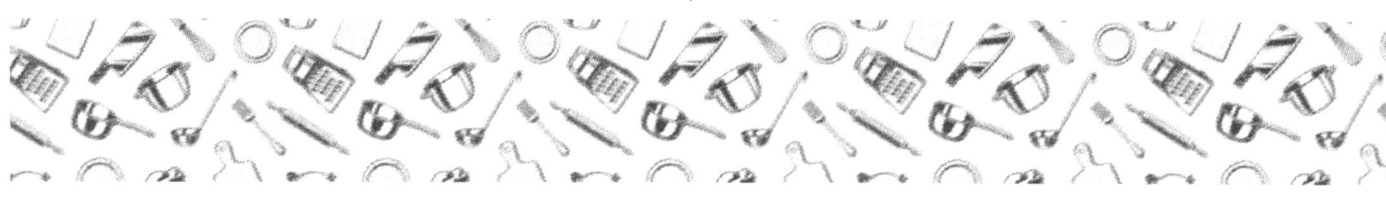

INGREDIENTS

2 tablespoons olive oil
4 (3.5 ounce) links sweet Italian sausage
1/2-pound cubed flank steak
8 links pork sausage
3 onion, chopped
5 cloves garlic, minced
2 (6 ounce) cans tomato paste
2 (28 ounce) cans crushed tomatoes
2 bay leaves
1 pinch ground cinnamon salt to taste
ground black pepper to taste
2 pounds lean ground beef
2 eggs
4 slices white bread, slice into cubes
1/2 cup grated Romano cheese
salt to taste
ground black pepper to taste
1 pinch dried parsley
2 tablespoons olive oil
2 (16 ounce) packages macaroni

Nutritional Value: 456 calories per serving

DIRECTIONS

1. In a large stock pot, heat olive oil over medium heat. Add Italian sausage, beef chunks, sausage links, onion, and garlic: cook and stir until meat is thoroughly done. Stir in tomato paste, crushed tomatoes, bay leaves, and cinnamon. Season with salt and pepper to taste. Simmer sauce over low heat for 1 hour.
2. In a large bowl, Mix the ground chuck beef, eggs, bread, Romano cheese, salt and pepper, and a pinch of parsley flakes. Shape into golf ball size meatballs.
3. Pour olive oil into a large skillet. Add meatballs and cook over medium heat until lightly browned. Place meatballs in spaghetti sauce, and simmer for 1 1/2 to 2 hours.
4. Cook pasta in boiling, salted water until al dente. Drain well, and transfer to a large bowl. Stir 1 cup sauce into the noodles to help prevent sticking.
5. Serve sauce with meatballs over pasta.

Pasta

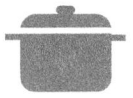

Pizza Pie Pasta

COOKING: 25 MIN   SERVES: 2

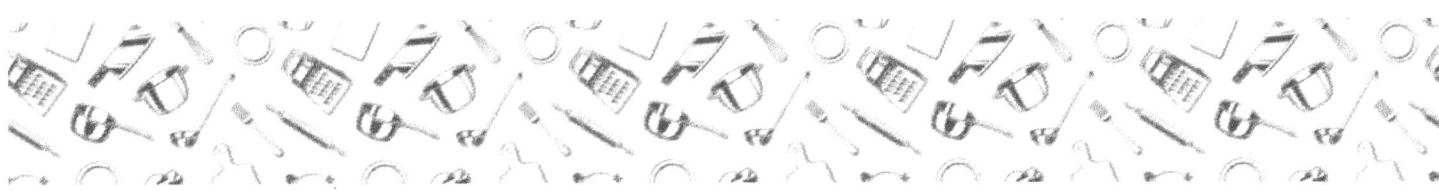

INGREDIENTS

1 tablespoon olive oil
1 large onion, chopped
1 cup sliced mushrooms Vegetable cooking spray
1 egg, beaten
1/4 cup milk
3 1/2 cups cooked tricolor or plain corkscrew-shaped pasta
1 cup shredded part-skim mozzarella cheese
1 1/2 cups Italian sauce

Nutritional Value: 436 calories per serving

DIRECTIONS

1. Heat oil in large skillet over medium heat. Add onion and mushrooms and cook until tender and almost all liquid is evaporated. Remove from heat. Spray 12-inch pizza pan with cooking spray.
2. Mix egg, milk, pasta and 1/2 cup cheese. Spread pasta mixture in an even layer on prepared pan.
3. Bake at 350 degrees F for 20 minutes.
4. Spread pasta sauce over pasta crust. Top with onion mixture. Sprinkle with remaining cheese. Bake for 18 minutes or until cheese is melted and sauce is hot. Let stand 5 minutes.

Would you like to become a master at chess and use all the best strategies availa[ble to] win every game?

Do you want your opponent to taste defeat?

Then keep reading...

This Step-By-Step Guide will teach you everything you need to know to be able t[o play] chess easily, starting from the most basics information about openings skills, un[til the] top-class strategies and techniques used by professional players.

Thanks to this guide, you will also learn :

- Everything about the main basic openings principles
- How to defend an opening used by the opponent
- Be taken from basic to a higher level of the game
- Powerful tactics and strategies that bring wins every time
- The most essential tips and advice to develop optimal checkmates and s[urprise] your opponent!
- Realize how playing chess is an incredibly beneficial past time improving [your] intelligence and to practice brain exercises.

...And Much More!

A lot of people tend to think that learning and mastering this awesome sport is [too] time-consuming and difficult...

...But it's not if you are using the right guide.

You will be able to keep your brain active and trained, you will boost your creativity, [focus] and memory while playing an awesome game, so...

...What are you waiting for? Scroll to the top of the page and click the "BUY NOW" b[utton] because playing chess has never been easier!

www.ingramcontent.com/pod-product-compliance
Lightning Source LLC
Chambersburg PA
CBHW081352080526
44588CB00016B/2470